The Washington Manual® Internship Survival Guide

Second Edition

Written and Edited by

Grace A. Lin, MD
Former Washington University Medicine
    Resident
Instructor of Medicine
Washington University School of Medicine
St. Louis, Missouri

Tammy L. Lin, MD
Former Washington University Medicine
    Resident
Assistant Clinical Professor of Medicine
University of California, San Diego
San Diego, California

Kaori A. Sakurai, MD
Former Washington University Medicine
    Resident
Private Practice
St. Louis, Missouri

Executive Editor
Thomas M. DeFer, MD
Former Washington University Medicine
    Resident
Assistant Professor of Internal Medicine
Washington University School of Medicine
St. Louis, Missouri

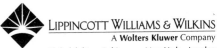
LIPPINCOTT WILLIAMS & WILKINS
A **Wolters Kluwer** Company
Philadelphia • Baltimore • New York • London
Buenos Aires • Hong Kong • Sydney • Tokyo

Acquisitions Editor: *Danette Somers*
Managing Editor: *Lauren Aquino*
Project Manager: *Nicole Walz*
Senior Manufacturing Manager: *Ben Rivera*
Senior Marketing Manager: *Kathleen Neely*
Design Coordinator: *Holly Reid McLaughlin*
Cover Design: *QT Design*
Production Services: *Maryland Composition Inc*
Printer: *RR Donnelley & Sons*

Library of Congress Cataloging-in-Publication Data

The Washington manual internship survival guide / written and edited by
Grace A. Lin, Tammy L. Lin, Kaori A. Sakurai ; executive editor,
Thomas M. Defer.—2nd ed.
    p. ; cm.
  Includes bibliographical references and index.
  ISBN 0-7817-8645-2
  1. Internal medicine—Handbooks, manuals, etc. 2. Interns (Medicine)—
Handbooks, manuals, etc. I. Title: Manual internship survival guide. II. Lin,
Grace A. III. Lin, Tammy L. IV Sakurai, Kaori A. V. DeFer, Thomas M.
VI. Washington
  [DNLM: 1. Internal Medicine—Handbooks. 2. Internship and
Residency—Handbooks. WB 39
W317 2006] University (Saint Louis, Mo.)
RC55.L56 2006
616—dc22

                                                            2005026134

Preface and Acknowledgments

This is the second edition of the highly successful, pocket sized companion "survival guide" written and edited by former Washington University residents. It is meant to be complementary to the *Washington Manual®* of *Medical Therapeutics* and the *Washington Manual®* of *Ambulatory Therapeutics* and to contain concise and practical information for those learning the basics of practicing clinical medicine. It is written assuming knowledge of basic pathophysiology and data interpretation. The target audience is primarily those beginning their internship, but this guide may be useful for medical students, residents, and anyone else on the front lines of patient care.

The second edition has been updated to be consistent with the most current medical practices, and several sections have been expanded, most notably the critical care section. In keeping with the purpose of a pocket book, a deliberate attempt was made to keep the format succinct so that common work-ups, cross-cover calls, procedures, and other practical information would always be in a rapidly accessible format. There are also essential sections about "what not to miss" and "when to call for help" for common clinical scenarios. It is written assuming that a standard textbook of internal medicine, the *Washington Manuals®*, a *Sanford Guide*, *Physicians Desk Reference*, and internet access (as well as your resident) are available nearby for reference.

We wish to thank the following members of the internal medicine residency program at Washington University for their thoughtful comments and suggestions that have made our guide immeasurably better: Robert Blanton, MD, Walter Chan, MD, Skye Chen, MD, Bryan Faller, MD, Shaila Gogate, MD, Christina Ha, MD, Ian Harris, MD, Sandeep Hindupur, MD, Christopher Holley, MD, Susan Holley, MD, Claire Kenneally, MD, Sakib Khalid, MD, David Lo, MD, Sam Lubner, MD, Leticia Luz, MD, Steven McEldowney, MD, Matthew Morrell, MD, Stephanie Park, MD, John Phillips, MD, Hilary Reno, MD, Jason Ricci, MD, Daniel Ringold, MD, Katherine Tsai, MD, Arun Varadhachary, MD, Deepak Voora, MD, Amy Wang, MD, and Patrick Win, MD.

We wish to thank Daniel Goodenberger, MD, and Kenneth Polonsky, MD, whose leadership and support have been instrumental to the continued success of this book. We wish to thank Lauren Aquino, Mary Choi, Kathy Neely, Nicole Walz, and Danette Somers from Lippincott, and Heidi Pongratz from Maryland Composition for their assistance. Finally, we wish to thank our families for their love and support, especially Ian Harris, Brian Kearns, and George, Jean, and Alice Lin.

Contributing Authors

These authors were all residents or faculty at Washington University at the time of their contributions. Some authors have since moved on to other positions

Dermatology:
Theresa Schroeder, MD
Dermatology Resident
Barnes-Jewish Hospital
St. Louis, Missouri

Michael Heffernan, MD
Assistant Professor of Dermatology
Barnes-Jewish Hospital
St. Louis, Missouri
Faculty Advisor

Medical Consultation:
Geoffrey Cislo, MD
Former Medical Chief Resident
Barnes-Jewish Hospital
St. Louis, Missouri

Michael Lazarus, MD
Former Medical Chief Resident
Barnes-Jewish Hospital
St. Louis, Missouri

Neurology:
Stephen Lee, MD
Neurology Resident
Barnes-Jewish Hospital
St. Louis, Missouri

Richard Sohn, MD
Professor of Neurology
Barnes-Jewish Hospital
St. Louis, Missouri
Faculty Advisor

Obstetrics and Gynecology:
Solange Wyatt, MD
Obstetrics and Gynecology Resident
Barnes-Jewish Hospital
St. Louis, Missouri

David Cohn, MD
Assistant Professor of Obstetrics
and Gynecology
Barnes-Jewish Hospital
St. Louis, Missouri
Faculty Advisor

Ophthalmology:
Samir Sayegh, MD
Ophthalmology Resident
Barnes-Jewish Hospital
St. Louis, Missouri

Jonathon Silbert, MD
Assistant Professor of
Ophthalmology and Visual
Sciences
Barnes-Jewish Hospital
St. Louis, Missouri
Faculty Advisor

Otolaryngology:
Christopher Yian, MD
Otolaryngology Resident
Barnes-Jewish Hospital
St. Louis, Missouri

Mark Wallace, MD
Assistant Professor of
Otolaryngology
Barnes-Jewish Hospital
St. Louis, Missouri
Faculty Advisor

Psychiatry:
David Montani, MD
Fellow, Forensic Psychiatry
Former Psychiatry Chief Resident
Chicago, Illinois

CONTRIBUTING AUTHORS

Radiology:
Ronald Gerstle, MD
Radiology Resident
Mallinkrodt Institute of Radiology
Barnes-Jewish Hospital
St. Louis, Missouri

General Surgery:
Ernerst Franklin, MD, MBA
General Surgery Resident
Barnes-Jewish Hospital
St. Louis, Missouri

Gerard Doherty, MD
Professor of Surgery
Barnes-Jewish Hospital
St. Louis, Missouri
Faculty Advisor

Orthopaedic Surgery:
Raja Dhalla, MD
Orthopaedic Surgery Resident
Barnes-Jewish Hospital
St. Louis, Missouri

David Miller, MD
Associate Professor of Orthopaedic
  Surgery
Barnes-Jewish Hospital
St. Louis, Missouri
Faculty Advisor

Internal Medicine:
John M. Mohart, MD
Internal Medicine Resident
Barnes-Jewish Hospital
St. Louis, Missouri

Abbreviations List

AAA	abdominal aortic aneurysm
AMA	against medical advice
AP	anteroposterior
APC	atrial premature contraction
ARF	acute renal failure
ATN	acute tubular necrosis
AVNRT	AV nodal reentrant tachycardia
AVRT	atrioventricular reciprocating tachycardia
BBB	bundle branch block
BP	bullous pemphigoid
CAD	coronary artery disease
CHF	congestive heart failure
COPD	chronic obstructive pulmonary disease
CPAP	continuous positive airway pressure
CXR	chest x-ray
D/C	discharge
DKA	diabetic ketoacidosis
ECF	extracellular fluid
FFP	fresh frozen plasma
GERD	gastroesophageal reflux disease
GN	glomerulonephritis
H&P	history and physical examination
β-hCG	human chorionic gonadotropin-β
Hct	hematocrit
HEENT	head, eyes, ears, nose, and throat
HTN	hypertension
I/O	input/output
JPCs	junctional premature contractions
JVP	jugular venous pressure
LBBB	left bundle branch block
LMWH	low-molecular-weight heparin
LP	lumbar puncture
LVH	left ventricular hypertrophy
NS	normal saline
NSAID	nonsteroidal antiinflammatory drug
NSR	normal sinus rhythm
PA	posteroanterior
PE	physical examination
PICC	peripherally inserted central catheter
PID	pelvic inflammatory disease

ABRREVIATIONS LIST

PUD	peptic ulcer disease
PV	pemphigus vulgaris
PVC	premature ventricular contraction
RR	respiratory rate
RTA	renal tubular acidosis
SBO	small bowel obstruction
SBP	systolic BP
SJS	Stevens-Johnson syndrome
SOB	shortness of breath
T	temperature
TDP	torsades de pointes
TIA	transient ischemic attack
TSH	thyroid-stimulating hormone
TSS	toxic shock syndrome
UTI	urinary tract infection
VPC	ventricular premature contraction

Contents

CONTENTS

CONTENTS

1 Keys to Survival

... Or how not *to get voted off of the island ...*

1. Don't panic.

2. Take care of your patients. You are finally using your education and training.

3. Be kind to the nurses and other ancillary staff. They can make your life much better ... or much worse.

4. Sleep when you can.

5. Remember to eat.

6. Wear comfortable shoes.

7. Call your significant other when on-call.

8. Verify everything (labs, x-rays, ECGs, etc.) yourself.

9. Ask questions and ask for help. Believe it or not, you are not expected to know everything.

10. Call for consultations on your patients early in the day and have a specific question you want answered from the consultant. This is always appreciated.

11. Start thinking about discharge/disposition planning from day 1.

12. Dictate discharge summaries the day the patient leaves.

13. When generating a differential diagnosis, look for an etiology in VITAMIN E:

    *V*ascular, *I*nfection/*I*nflammatory, *T*rauma, *A*cquired/ *A*utoimmune, *M*etabolic/*M*edications, *I*nherited/*I*atrogenic/ *I*diopathic, *N*eoplastic, *E*nvironmental

14. Work hard, stay enthusiastic, and maintain interest!

2 ACLS Algorithms

... First, take a deep breath. Second, take your own pulse. Now you can begin worrying about the patient ...

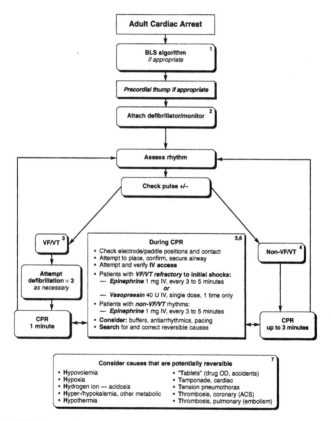

FIGURE 2-1. ILCOR Universal/International ACLS Algorithm. (From Guidelines 2000 for cardiopulmonary resuscitation and emergency cardiovascular care. Part 6: advanced cardiovascular life support: 7C: a guide to the international ACLS algorithms. The American Heart Association in collaboration with the International Liaison Committee on Resuscitation. *Circulation* 2000;102[Suppl 8]:I-143, with permission.)

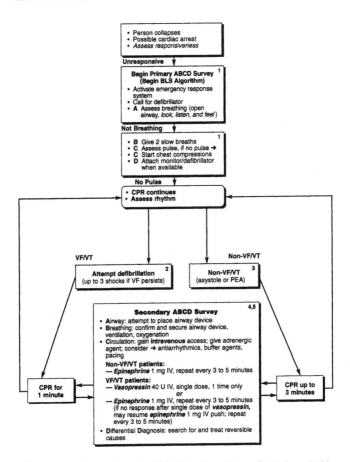

FIGURE 2-2. Comprehensive ECC Algorithm. (From Guidelines 2000 for cardiopulmonary resuscitation and emergency cardiovascular care. Part 6: advanced cardiovascular life support: 7C: a guide to the International ACLS algorithms. The American Heart Association in collaboration with the International Liaison Committee on Resuscitation. *Circulation* 2000;102[Suppl 8]:I-144, with permission.)

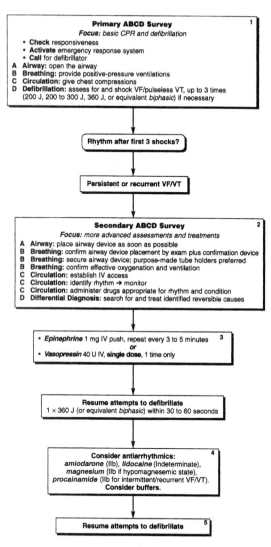

Primary ABCD Survey   1
Focus: basic CPR and defibrillation
- **Check** responsiveness
- **Activate** emergency response system
- **Call** for defibrillator
A **Airway:** open the airway
B **Breathing:** provide positive-pressure ventilations
C **Circulation:** give chest compressions
D **Defibrillation:** assess for and shock VF/pulseless VT, up to 3 times (200 J, 200 to 300 J, 360 J, or equivalent *biphasic*) if necessary

Rhythm after first 3 shocks?

Persistent or recurrent VF/VT

Secondary ABCD Survey   2
Focus: more advanced assessments and treatments
A **Airway:** place airway device as soon as possible
B **Breathing:** confirm airway device placement by exam plus confirmation device
B **Breathing:** secure airway device; purpose-made tube holders preferred
B **Breathing:** confirm effective oxygenation and ventilation
C **Circulation:** establish IV access
C **Circulation:** identify rhythm → monitor
C **Circulation:** administer drugs appropriate for rhythm and condition
D **Differential Diagnosis:** search for and treat identified reversible causes

- *Epinephrine* 1 mg IV push, repeat every 3 to 5 minutes   3
or
- *Vasopressin* 40 U IV, **single dose,** 1 time only

Resume attempts to defibrillate
1 × 360 J (or equivalent *biphasic*) within 30 to 60 seconds

Consider antiarrhythmics: 4
amiodarone (IIb), *lidocaine* (Indeterminate),
magnesium (IIb if hypomagnesemic state),
procainamide (IIb for intermittent/recurrent VF/VT).
Consider buffers.

Resume attempts to defibrillate   5

FIGURE 2-3. Ventricular Fibrillation/Pulseless VT Algorithm. (From Guidelines 2000 for cardiopulmonary resuscitation and emergency cardiovascular care. Part 6: advanced cardiovascular life support: 7C: a guide to the International ACLS algorithms. The American Heart Association in collaboration with the International Liaison Committee on Resuscitation. *Circulation* 2000;102[Suppl 8]:I-147, with permission.)

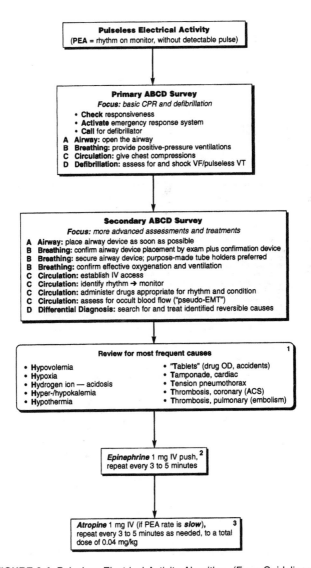

FIGURE 2-4. Pulseless Electrical Activity Algorithm. (From Guidelines 2000 for cardiopulmonary resuscitation and emergency cardiovascular care. Part 6: advanced cardiovascular life support: 7C: a guide to the International ACLS algorithms. The American Heart Association in collaboration with the International Liaison Committee on Resuscitation. *Circulation* 2000;102[Suppl 8]:I-151, with permission.)

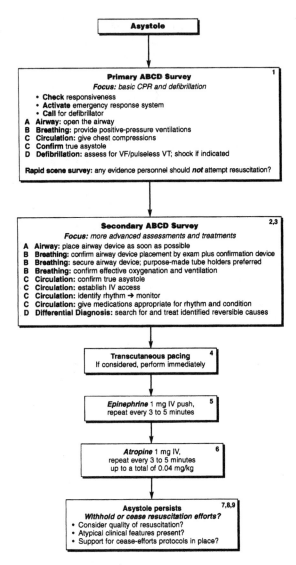

FIGURE 2-5. Asystole: The Silent Heart Algorithm. (From Guidelines 2000 for cardiopulmonary resuscitation and emergency cardiovascular care. Part 6: advanced cardiovascular life support: 7C: a guide to the International ACLS algorithms. The American Heart Association in collaboration with the International Liaison Committee on Resuscitation. *Circulation* 2000;102[Suppl 8]:I-153, with permission.)

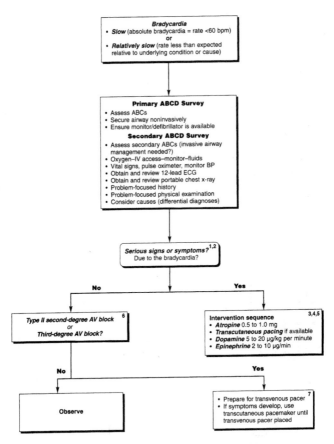

FIGURE 2-6. Bradycardia Algorithm. (From Guidelines 2000 for cardiopulmonary resuscitation and emergency cardiovascular care. Part 6: advanced cardiovascular life support: 7C: a guide to the International ACLS algorithms. The American Heart Association in collaboration with the International Liaison Committee on Resuscitation. *Circulation* 2000;102[Suppl 8]:I-156, with permission.)

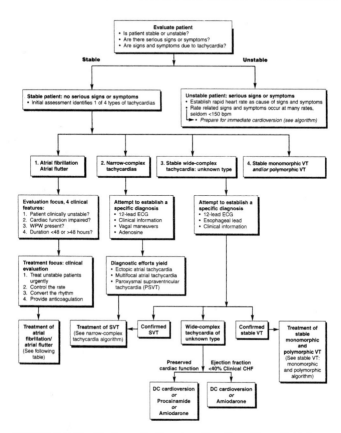

FIGURE 2-7. The Tachycardia Overview Algorithm. (From Guidelines 2000 for cardiopulmonary resuscitation and emergency cardiovascular care. Part 6: advanced cardiovascular life support: 7D: the tachycardia algorithms. The American Heart Association in collaboration with the International Liaison Committee on Resuscitation. *Circulation* 2000; 102[Suppl 8]:I-159, with permission.)

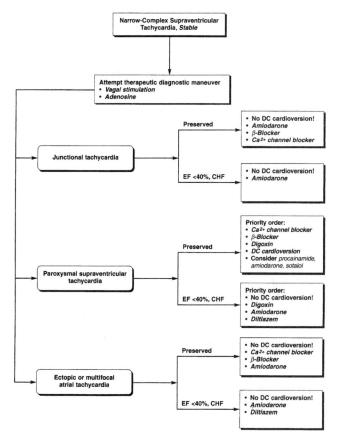

FIGURE 2-8. Narrow Complex Supraventricular Tachycardia Algorithm. (From Guidelines 2000 for cardiopulmonary resuscitation and emergency cardiovascular care. Part 6: advanced cardiovascular life support: 7D: the tachycardia algorithms. The American Heart Association in collaboration with the International Liaison Committee on Resuscitation. *Circulation* 2000;102[Suppl 8]:I-162, with permission.)

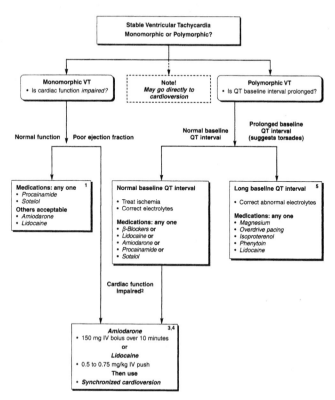

FIGURE 2-9. Stable Ventricular Tachycardia (Monomorphic or Polymorphic) Algorithm. (From Guidelines 2000 for cardiopulmonary resuscitation and emergency cardiovascular care. Part 6: advanced cardiovascular life support: 7D: the tachycardia algorithms. The American Heart Association in collaboration with the International Liaison Committee on Resuscitation. *Circulation* 2000;102[Suppl 8]:I-163, with permission.)

3

Accumulating Your War Chest

... The best defense is a good offense ...

BOOKS AND TOOLS TO CARRY WITH YOU

Most house officers carry a compact general manual of internal medicine in their pocket. Any of the following are useful and practical:

- Green G, Harris I, Lin G, Moylan K, eds. *The Washington Manual of Medical Therapeutics*, 31st ed. Lippincott Williams & Wilkins, 2004.

- Cheng A, Zaas A, McKusick V, eds. *The Osler Medical Handbook.* Mosby, 2003.

- Ferri FF, ed. *Practical Guide to the Care of the Medical Patient*, 6th ed. Mosby, 2004.

- Gomella LG, Haist SA. *Clinician's Pocket Reference,* 10th ed. McGraw-Hill Medical, 2003.

- Huang ES, Tang WH, Lee DS, Thomason CC, Fischer MA. *Internal Medicine: Handbook for Clinicians.* Scrub-Hill Press, 2000.

- Sabatine, M. *Pocket Medicine.* Lippincott Williams & Wilkins, 2004.

- Dubin D, ed. *Rapid Interpretation of EKG's*, 6th ed. Cover Publishing Company, 2000. (Okay, so it's not likely that you're going to carry this around with you, but it's a great resource to keep in your locker or backpack.)

Other small pocket guides you don't want to be without:

- *Tarascon Pocket Pharmacopoeia.* Tarascon Publishing. Updated yearly.

- Winshall J, Lederman R. *Tarascon Internal Medicine and Critical Care Pocketbook, 3rd ed.* Tarascon Publishing, 2004.

- Rollings RC, Erica T, eds. *Facts and Formulas.* McNaughton & Gunn, 1984.

- Gilbert DN, Moellering RC, Sande MA, eds. *The Sanford Guide to Antimicrobial Therapy.* Antimicrobial Therapy Inc. Updated yearly.

Other things to carry with you:

- A good stethoscope

- Reflex hammer

- Guaiac developer and stool cards
- Penlight
- ECG calipers
- Ophthalmoscope/otoscope (Yes, you still need this; make sure it's charged for your call and leave it in your locker.)
- ABG kit
- Alcohol wipes
- Notecards for patient information

HANDHELD COMPUTER RESOURCES

... All in the palm of your hand ...

Drug References

- ePocrates   www.epocrates.com   Free (basic program)/$.
- Tarascon Pocket Pharmacopoeia   www.tarascon.com $.

Calculators

- MedMath   http://smi-web.stanford.edu/people/pcheng/medmath   Free.
- MedCalc   www.med-ia.ch/medcalc   Free.
- ABGPro   www.stacworks.com   Free.
- Archimedes   www.skyscape.com   Free.
- ICU Math   www.freewarepalm.com/medical/icumath.shtml   Free.
- PainSTAT   www.goldenratiodesign.com   Free.

Data Tracking

- Patient Keeper   www.patientkeeper.com $.
- Patient Tracker   www.handheldmed.com $.
- ePatient   www.iatrosoft.com $.
- WardWatch   www.watch.aust.com/pilot/wardwatch $.

Other References

- The Sanford Guide to Antimicrobial Therapy   www.sanfordguide.com $.
- Hopkins Antibiotic Guide   http://hopkins-abxguide.org   Free.
- STATcoder (several guidelines/calculators)   www.statcoder.com   Free.

- Medical Eponyms   http://eponyms.net   Free.
- Journal to Go (journal abstracts and news stories) www.journaltogo.com   Free.
- Diagnosaurus (differential diagnoses) http://books.mcgraw-hill.com/medical/diagnosaurus/index.html Free.

Other Useful Sites

- Skyscape Products   www.skyscape.com   Free (some stuff)/$.

The home of Harrison's, the Washington Manual, 5 Minute Clinical Consult (all are for purchase).

- Avantgo   www.avantgo.com   Free.

Download great web sites to your PalmPilot.

- PDA MD   www.pdamd.com   Free.

Comprehensive site with news reviews, columns, forums, tutorials, and products.

- Ectopic Brain   http://pbrain.hypermart.net   Free.

Comprehensive site dedicated to use of PDAs in clinical practice. Includes tips, product reviews, and links to sites for downloading useful products.

- Freeware for Palm or Freeware4PC   www.freewarepalm.com or www.freeware4pc.com   Free.

Database of available freeware for handhelds

- Your institution's house staff homepage may allow you to download useful things like pager numbers, e-mail addresses, and a weekly conference schedule.

INTERNET RESOURCES

… Unfortunately, sleep is not downloadable at this time …

General Sites

www.uptodate.com (UpToDate, $)
www.medscape.com (Medscape)
www.emedicine.com (eMedicine)
www.guideline.gov (National Guidelines Clearinghouse)
www.mdconsult.com (MD Consult; $)
www.acponline.org (American College of Physicians)

Cardiovascular Disease

www.nhlbi.nih.gov (National Heart, Lung, and Blood Institute)
www.acc.org (American College of Cardiology)

Cerebrovascular Disease and Stroke

www.ninds.nih.gov (National Institute of Neurological Diseases)
www.stroke.org (National Stroke Association)
www.strokecenter.org (Washington University)

Pulmonary Diseases and Allergy

www.chestnet.org (American College of Chest Physicians)

Endocrine and Diabetes

www.niddk.nih.gov (National Institute of Diabetes and Digestive and
    Kidney Diseases)
www.diabetes.org (American Diabetes Association)
www.endo-society.org (The Endocrine Society)
www.thyroid.org (American Thyroid Association)

Rheumatology

www.niams.nih.gov (National Institute of Arthritis and Musculoskele-
    tal and Skin Diseases)
www.rheumatology.org (American College of Rheumatology)

Nephrology

www.niddk.nih.gov (National Institute of Diabetes and Digestive and
    Kidney Diseases)
www.renalnet.org (RenalNet—Kidney Information Clearinghouse)
www.kidney.org (National Kidney Foundation)

Oncology

www.cancer.gov (National Cancer Institute)
www.nccn.org (National Comprehensive Cancer Network)

Orthopaedic Surgery

www.orthoinfo.aaos.org (American Association of Orthopaedic Sur-
    geons)

Gastroenterology

www.gastro.org (American Gastroenterological Association)
www.acg.gi.org (American College of Gastroenterology)

Infectious Disease/HIV

hivinsite.ucsf.edu (University of California at San Francisco—HIV
    site)
www.cdc.gov (Centers for Disease Control and Prevention)
www.niaid.nih.gov (National Institute of Allergy and Infectious Dis-
    eases)
www.who.int (World Health Organization)

Geriatrics, Aging, Osteoporosis

www.alzheimers.org (Alzheimer's Disease Education and Referral Center)
www.aoa.dhhs.gov (Administration on Aging)
www.osteo.org (National Institutes of Health—Osteoporosis and Related Bone Diseases-National Resource Center)

Complementary and Alternative Medicine

nccam.nih.gov (National Center for Complementary and Alternative Medicine)
www.nlm.nih.gov/medlineplus/herbalmedicine.html (Medline Plus)

Online Journals (subscriptions may be required)

www.annals.org (Annals of Internal Medicine)
www.bmj.com (British Medical Journal)
www.jama.ama-assn.org (Journal of the American Medical Association)
www.thelancet.com (The Lancet)
www.nejm.org (New England Journal of Medicine)

INTERNET RESOURCES FOR EVIDENCE-BASED MEDICINE

The Cochrane Database of Systematic Reviews

http://thecochranelibrary.net
Reviews, analyzes, and synthesizes the best clinical trials by topics.
Multi-directional links MEDLINE, EBM, and EUCLID full-text. Subscription required.

PubMed

www.nlm.nih.gov/entrez/query.fcgi
Maintained by the National Library of Medicine
Allows a user-friendly approach to medical literature with built-in search filters. Free.

ACP Journal Club

www.acpjc.org
Evidence-Based Medicine reviews of journal articles. Subscription required.

4 Useful Formulas

... CORRECTED SLEEP EQUATION ...

$$\text{Sleep (hrs)} = \frac{(\text{Discharges} + \text{Transfers})}{(\text{Admissions} + \text{Cross Cover})^2} \times \text{Interns}$$

A-a O$_2$ GRADIENT

A-a gradient = $PAo_2 - Pao_2$
Normal = $3-16$ (<8 if younger than 30 years old)

- $PAo_2 = (FIo_2 \times 713) - \left(\dfrac{PaCo_2}{0.8}\right)$

  Pao_2, Pco_2, and PAo_2 in mmHg

- Correction of gradient for age $2.5 + 0.25$ (age)

Causes of Increased A-a Gradient

- $\dot{V}/\dot{Q}$ mismatch

- Intrapulmonary right-to-left shunt.

- Intracardiac right-to-left shunt.

- Impaired diffusion (room air only).

ANION GAP (SERUM)

$AG = [Na^+] - ([Cl^-] + [HCO_3])$

$[Na^+]$, $[Cl^-]$, $HCO_3]$ in meq/L

Normal = $8-12$ mEq/L
See Acid-Base section in Chapter 16 for differential diagnosis.

ANION GAP (URINE)

$UAG = (U[Na^+] + U[K^+]) - U[Cl^-]$

$U[Na^+]$, $U[K^+]$, $U[Cl^-]$ in meq/L

Normal = slightly positive

- UAG is **negative** in diarrhea-induced nongap metabolic acidosis (**enhanced** urinary NH_4 excretion).

- UAG is **positive** in distal RTA–induced nongap metabolic acidosis (**impaired** urinary NH_4 excretion).

BODY MASS INDEX

BMI $= Wt(kg)/(Ht(m))^2$
or

BMI $= [Wt (lbs)/(Ht (in))^2] \times 703$

<18.5, underweight.
18.5–24.9, normal weight.
25–29.9, overweight.
>30, obese.

CREATININE CLEARANCE
Estimated (Cockcroft–Gault Formula):

$$CrCl = \frac{(140 - age) \times weight}{Cr \times 72}$$

Multiply by 0.85 for women.
Weight in kilograms, creatinine in mg/dL

Measured:

$$CrCl = \frac{U[Cr] \times Uvolume}{P[Cr] \times time}$$

Creatinine in mg/dL, volume in mL, and time in minutes.
Normal CrCl >100 mL/min

CORRECTED SERUM CALCIUM

Corrected serum Ca = measured $[Ca^{+2}]$ + $[0.8 \times (4.0 -$ measured albumin)]
$[Ca^{+2}]$ in mg/dL, albumin in g/dL

CORRECTED SERUM SODIUM

Corrected serum Na = measured $[Na^+]$ + $[0.016 \times$ (measured [glucose] $-$ 100)]
$[Na^+]$ in meq/L, [glucose] in mg/dL

FRACTIONAL EXCRETION OF SODIUM

$$FENa = \frac{U[Na^+] \times P[Cr]}{P[Na^+] \times U[Cr]} \times 100$$

$U[Na^+]$ and $P[Na^+]$ in meq/L; $U[Cr]$ and $P[Cr]$ in mg/dL
FENa <1% in prerenal states; not valid when diuretics have been given.

FRACTIONAL EXCRETION OF UREA

$$FEurea = \frac{U[urea] \times P[Cr]}{BUN \times U[Cr]} \times 100$$

U[urea] and BUN in mg/dL; U[Cr] and P[Cr] in mg/dL
FEurea <35% in prerenal states; not affected by diuretics.

MEAN ARTERIAL PRESSURE

$$MAP = \frac{SBP + (2 \times DBP)}{3}$$

OSMOLALITY (SERUM, ESTIMATED)

Calculated serum osmolality =

$$(2 \times [Na^+]) + \frac{[glucose]}{18} + \frac{BUN}{2.8}$$

$[Na^+]$ in meq/L; [glucose] and [BUN] in mg/dL

OSMOLAL GAP

Osmolal gap = measured S_{osm} − calculated S_{osm}

Causes of Increased Osmolal Gap

• Decreased serum water

  Hyperproteinemia
  Hypertriglyceridemia

• Presence of unmeasured osmoles

  Sorbitol, glycerol, mannitol, ethanol, isopropyl alcohol, acetone, ethyl ether, methanol, and ethylene glycol

RETICULOCYTE COUNT (CORRECTED)

Corrected reticulocyte count =

$$\text{Observed reticulocyte count} \times \left(\frac{\text{Measured Hct \%}}{45 \%}\right)$$

RETICULOCYTE PRODUCTION INDEX

$$RPI = \frac{\text{Corrected reticulocyte count}}{\text{Maturation index}}$$

$$\text{Maturation index} = 1 + \left(0.5 \times \frac{(45\text{-Hct})}{10}\right)$$

• The reticulocyte count is not accurate in anemia, so use the reticulocyte production index.

• Good marrow response = 2.0–6.0.

MEDICAL EPIDEMIOLOGY

Test Result	Disease	No Disease
Positive	True positive (A)	False positive (B)
Negative	False negative (C)	True negative (D)

- **Sensitivity:** The percentage of patients with the target disorder who have a positive result (A/[A + C]). The greater the sensitivity, the more likely the test will detect patients with the disease. High sensitivity tests are useful clinically to rule OUT a disease (SnOUT) (i.e., a negative test result would virtually exclude the possibility of the disease).

- **Specificity:** The percentage of patients without the target disorder who have a negative test result (D/[B + D]). Very specific tests are used to confirm or rule IN the presence of disease (SpIN).

- **Positive predictive value (PPV):** The percentage of persons with positive test results who actually have the disease (A/[A + B]).

- **Negative predictive value (NPV):** The percentage of persons with negative test results in which the disease is absent (D/[C + D]).

- **Number needed to treat (NNT):** The number of patients who need to be treated to achieve one additional favorable outcome; calculated as 1/absolute risk reduction (ARR), rounded up to the nearest whole number.

- **Number needed to harm (NNH):** The number of patients who, if they received the experimental treatment, would lead to one additional person being harmed compared with patients who receive the control treatment; calculated as 1/absolute risk increase (ARI).

5 Triage

BEFORE ACCEPTING ADMISSIONS

... Do ask, do tell ...

1. Obtain vital stats: name, date of birth, medical record number, current location, and attending physician.

2. Why does the patient need to be admitted to your service?

3. Is the patient competent, and does he or she want to be admitted?

4. What are the patient's chief complaints, comorbidities, relevant past medical history, and brief history?

5. When was the last previous admission? Obtain old medical records (inpatient and outpatient).

6. Obtain vital signs, pertinent examination including mental status, key lab data, CXR, ECG, and code status. Review as many lab results and films in the ER as you can.

7. Confirm IV access.

8. Inquire about major interventions performed, medications given, and consultations pending.

9. What follow-up is necessary (i.e., lab tests that are pending, consults that need to be called, blood transfusions, antibiotics)?

10. Find out who the primary MD is and if this person has been notified.

11. Do family members need to be called?

OTHER IMPORTANT QUESTIONS TO CONSIDER

... Location, location, location ...

- Is this an appropriate admission for your service (i.e., Is there something you can do for the patient that no one else can do? Does a different service make more sense?)?

- Can this patient be managed as an outpatient? If yes, social services may need to be involved. In addition, arranging follow-up is crucial.

- Is the patient stable enough for the floors? Are any more treatments needed before transfer to the floor (i.e., nebulizer treatments, etc.)?

- Can your staff adequately handle this patient?

- What specific interventions does this patient need that other institutions cannot provide (in the case of a hospital-to-hospital transfer)?

- Obtain collateral information from family, nursing homes, or other caregivers. Always collect and hold on to important phone contacts.

6 Cross-Coverage

... Who? What? Wait, let me get my sign-out ...

GENERAL POINTS

1. For the first few months of residency, when you are called about a patient, it is a good idea to go see the patient and assess the situation. Do this until you feel comfortable deciding what situations can be adequately handled over the telephone with the nurses and the support staff.

2. Always go see the patient if you have any doubt or concern. The patient is always your number one priority.

3. If you do go see a patient, always write a note (this can be brief, depending on the situation). Things to document include

   A. Reason you were called to see patient (i.e., CTSP for chest pain).

   B. Assessment of situation on arrival including general appearance, vitals, pertinent physical examination.

   C. Interventions.

   D. Outcome.

REASONS YOU MUST GO SEE A PATIENT

... Drop everything and go now. Godspeed ...

1. Any major changes in clinical status.

   - Altered mental status or other changes in neurologic state.
   - Dyspnea.
   - Chest pain.
   - Severe abdominal pain.
   - Seizures.
   - Uncontrolled bleeding (hemoptysis, hematemesis, lower GI bleed, hematuria, vaginal bleeding).
   - Uncontrolled vomiting.
   - Severe headache.
   - New onset of pain.
   - Falls.

2. Any major changes in vital signs.

- Oxygen desaturation.

- Hypotension.

- Arrhythmias (tachyarrhythmias and bradyarrhythmias).

- Fever associated with changes in mental status, changes in vital signs.

THINGS TO CONSIDER ASKING FOR BEFORE ARRIVAL AT BEDSIDE

... Delegate before it's too late ...

1. Full set of vitals.

2. Hospital chart at bedside.

3. IV access.

4. Oxygen (nasal cannula, face mask), respiratory therapist.

5. Cardiac monitor, ECG.

6. Crash/code cart.

7. Chest x-ray.

8. ABG kits.

9. Blood cultures, if febrile.

10. Basic lab results.

11. Restraints.

12. In situations in which the patient is becoming unstable and you are having difficulty, have the resident paged immediately!

THINGS THAT CAN WAIT

... Passing back the pain ...

1. Talking to family members; unless urgent, this can usually be handled by the primary team.

2. Major adjustments in medication regimen in a stable patient (i.e., diabetic medicines, antihypertensive medicines, antibiotics).

3. Consultations in nonemergent, stable situations (i.e., GI consult in patient with Hemoccult-positive brown stool, stable hematocrit, stable vital signs).

4. Renewal of restraints/telemetry orders.

5. Addressing code status in a stable patient.

APPROPRIATE TRANSFER OF PATIENTS TO THE INTENSIVE CARE UNIT

... Passing on the pain ...

1. Determine which unit is most appropriate for management of the patient.

2. Speak to the resident who will be accepting the patient to inform him or her of the situation.

3. Have the nursing staff give report to the staff in the unit.

4. Every patient needs a brief transfer note, including:

    A. When and why you were called to see the patient.

    B. One-line description of patient and his or her comorbidities.

    C. Your assessment of the situation.

    D. Your management of the situation, including diagnostic and therapeutic measures, complications, and outcome. Include code note, if appropriate.

    E. Your assessment and plan at this point with brief differential diagnosis of what could be going on.

    F. Reason for transfer (pressors, arrhythmias, unstable vital signs, closer monitoring, etc.).

    G. Code status.

    H. Who has been notified (patient's physician, family members).

7 Patient and Staff Relations

... It's like winking in the dark, you know what you're doing, but make sure everyone else does, too ...

WORKING WITH ANCILLARY STAFF

- Give specific directions and use your judgment, but also give others a chance to make suggestions and solve problems. Effective use of ancillary staff can greatly increase your efficiency.

- A compliment for a job well done goes a long way (others are overworked, too), and you will be remembered when you need help.

- Criticize in private. Constructive feedback may be necessary and welcomed if done in a nonjudgmental manner.

- Regard ancillary staff as fellow members of the patient care team; they are often "bothering" you out of concern for the patient and not to harass you.

- Efforts to let team members know the plan can save you phone calls and increase sleep.

REFERRING A PATIENT

- When referring a patient to the ER, another physician, or transferring a patient, always make a courtesy call first.

- Pertinent information includes:
  1. Who you are.
  2. Patient identification information.
  3. Succinct history of the problem.
  4. Supporting lab data.
  5. Suggestions for further evaluation.
  6. Likely disposition of the patient.
  7. A contact number where you or someone covering for you can be reached for questions or follow-up information.

WORKING WITH DIFFICULT PATIENTS

... Having fun yet? ...

- Be proactive and address potential concerns, expectations, or questions up front. Checking in with the patient at regular intervals builds rapport and can save you from multiple phone calls. Try to minimize waiting time and interruptions during meetings.

- Be as flexible and as accommodating as you can. Recognize that the patient may be tired of repeating his or her history or having a physical examination.

- Let the patient (and loved ones) know about the management plan at least once a day. Follow up with them on test results and changes in the plan, and let them know if consultants will be coming by.

- If more than one service is involved, designate someone to be the primary source of communication to avoid confusion.

- The patient's ''difficult'' behavior may stem from lack of control over decision making and the situation or lack of insight into his or her medical condition. Past experiences, things the patient may have seen or read in the media, and fear may also play a role. *Active* listening, acknowledging the patient's point of view, and reassurance can go a long way.

- Acknowledge your own frustration, seek the advice of others when necessary, and always try to do what's best for the patient.

TABLE 7-1.
POTENTIAL RESOURCES AND OPTIONS

Resources	Options
Nursing supervisor or manager	Individual or joint meetings with or without loved ones (useful for any situation below).
Social worker	Initial evaluation for nursing home, rehab, or extended care facility placement.
Case coordinator	Return to nursing home issues; durable medical equipment; insurance disputes and concerns. Home health/home infusion/hospice referrals. Transportation issues.
Risk management	For litigious patients/family members, if you have concerns about the case, or if you expect a poor outcome.
Ombudsman or ethics committee	Helpful if there are disputes between physicians or family members.
Family members or loved ones	Proceed cautiously; if there are family members who are in disagreement, try to remain neutral.
Religious resources	For spiritual support and issues related to death and end of life.
A new physician	A new physician may be the best solution if other options have failed.

TABLE 7-2.
DEALING WITH DIFFICULT PROBLEMS

Problem	Suggestions	Potential Actions
Abuses of the system (i.e., narcotics)	Set boundaries; written contracts are often helpful (be specific in stating the problem and plan).	Notify all members of the team caring for the patient.
		Document concisely in the chart and include on sign out.
Manipulative patients	See above.	See above.
	Coordinate care through one team member to maintain consistency.	
Violent patients (see Chap. 17, Psychiatry section)	*Safety first.*	See above.
	Tell others you are seeing the patient. Try to remain calm and neutral.	Contact security or law enforcement officials if necessary.
	Always stand between the patient and the door.	Arrange to have security nearby when you see the patient.
	Remove all potentially dangerous items that can be used against you (i.e., stethoscope).	
Patients who want to leave AMA	First, establish competence (see Psychiatry Consultation section, Chap. 17).	See above.
		Have patient sign AMA form.
	Then, listen to the patient's reason(s).	Carefully document discussion of risks and benefits in the chart.
	Respond in a nondefensive, nonjudgmental manner.	Try to arrange discharge medications and follow-up plans.
	Calmly explain the risks and consequences of leaving.	Advise the patient to seek medical attention again if condition worsens.
	Explain the benefits of staying and the importance of completing the diagnostic/treatment plan.	Notify the attending of record of AMA discharge.
	Be accommodating if possible.	
	Enlist the help of other team/family members.	

(Continued)

TABLE 7-2.
DEALING WITH DIFFICULT PROBLEMS (Continued)

Problem	Suggestions	Potential Actions
Homelessness or return to abusive situations	Social work is a helpful resource.	Refer patients to local shelters or to local shelters/safe havens.
		Contact proper authorities (i.e., police, Division of Aging, Child and Family Services).
		Careful, neutral documentation in the medical record.
Refusal of nursing home placement	Social work, family members, and other team members can assist and discuss with patient.	Emphasize that it may be a temporary stay.
	Consider rehabilitation as a potential place for referral.	Try to arrange for close out-patient follow-up, home health services, and other family members to check in and help.
		Ultimately, you may have to respect the patient's wishes.
High likelihood that patient will abuse substances again	Consider chemical dependency consult.	Educate the patient on hazards of substance abuse.
		Consider inpatient or out-patient follow-up.
Concern for suicide or homicide (see Chap. 17, Psychiatry section)	Consider psychiatry consultation, assess competency.	Document carefully in the chart.
		Place patient on suicide precautions with sitter.
		Consider possible transfer to inpatient psychiatric setting

(*Continued*)

TABLE 7-2.
DEALING WITH DIFFICULT PROBLEMS (Continued)

Problem	Suggestions	Potential Actions
Financial difficulties	Social workers or case co-ordinators can be very helpful.	Notify family members and loved ones.
		Payment and transportation arrangements can be made.
		Medication samples.
		Referral to free clinics and resources.
		Assistance with applying for Medicaid, disability, etc.

TABLE 7-3.
ADDRESSING END-OF-LIFE ISSUES

Issue	Suggestions
Code status Intubation CPR Vasopressors Cardioversion Antibiotics and other medications Nutrition (i.e., G-tubes) Phlebotomy IV lines Withdrawal of support Comfort care	Explain it in language and terms the patient and family members can understand. Remain neutral, although it is appropriate to give your opinion, especially if asked. Be very specific and clear (i.e., the exact interventions to be done or not to be done) in your discussion and **document clearly in the medical record.** **Communicate status with other team members.** Give sufficient time to consider the decision, and explain this decision can be changed. Be open and available for further discussion and questions. If patient is not able to discuss this with you, contact primary physician and family members, power of attorney.

8

Admissions

$$\text{Admission Pain Index (Harris index)} = \frac{\text{Patient's age (years)} \times \text{Length of stay (days)}}{\text{Glasgow Coma Scale score}}$$

GENERAL POINTS

1. When called with a new admission, it is critical to review old records, lab results, and old charts. However, if the patient is accessible, always eyeball the patient first and check vital signs before digging through old records. With that said, old records are invaluable. Most systems have old lab results, discharge summaries, and H & Ps stored as electronic versions; use these extensively, but always confirm with your own eyes and ears.

2. After assessment of the patient and examination, admission orders should be completed as soon as possible. This will help the nursing staff and will enable you to get appropriate lab results in a timely manner. If you need stat labs, always inform the nursing staff directly. It is also helpful to inform the nurses when your orders are complete. Telemetry orders should also be completed as soon as possible if needed.

3. The history and physical examination should be well engrained by now. It is often helpful to dictate the H & P right after evaluating the patient. If you decide to dictate, you must ensure that a signed copy of the dictation makes it into the medical record chart. A short handwritten note of the current admission problems and short assessment should also be entered in the chart while awaiting the dictated H & P. Lab results can be added manually to the dictation as an addendum.

4. If the patient has a private primary care physician, he or she should be notified as soon as possible regarding the admission, and your plan should be communicated to the private physician. Many private physicians or their covering partners like to be notified as soon as possible, regardless of the time of night.

5. In summary, remember the three pearls of an admission:
   - Assess the stability of the patient: *Do this first.*

   - Obtain a good H & P, even if this has already been done by another medical team.

- Write orders as soon as possible. This makes the nurses and unit clerks happy and allows you to get the lab data you need to finish your evaluation.

ADMISSION ORDERS

Many admission diagnoses have preset clinical pathways and associated order sets (i.e., CHF, asthma). These are often helpful. Also, consider the patient's eligibility for appropriate research studies.
The mnemonic ADCVAANDISML may be useful.

Admit to ward/attending/house officers.

Diagnosis.

Condition.

Vitals: e.g., routine, every shift, every 2 hours. Always include call orders (i.e., call HO for SBP >180 or <90, pulse >130 or <60, RR >30 or <10, T >38.3°C, O_2 saturation <92%).

Allergies and reactions.

Activity (ad lib, bedrest with bedside commode, up to chair, etc.).

Nursing (strict I/O, daily weights, guaiac stools, Accuchecks, Foleys, etc.).

Diet (NPO, prudent diabetic, low fat/low cholesterol, renal, low salt, etc.).

IV (IV fluids, heplock).

Special (wound care, consults with social work, dietitian, and PT/OT).

Meds: All medications should include dosage, timing, route, and indications. Don't forget prn meds or you will be called often; if no contraindications, include acetaminophen (Tylenol), bisacodyl (Dulcolax) or docusate (Colace), and aluminum and magnesium hydroxide (Maalox).

Laboratory (don't forget to include a.m. labs).

Don't forget DVT prophylaxis for every patient who is not ambulating and GI prophylaxis for critically ill patients (see below for guidelines)!

DVT PROPHYLAXIS

- Indications: Patients with one or more risk factors and confined to bed; critical care patients.

- Risk factors for DVT: Cardiac dysfunction (heart failure, arrhythmia, MI), malignancy, surgery, trauma (especially orthopedic), previous DVT, obesity, smoking, age >40 yrs, inflammatory disease (e.g., inflammatory bowel disease, lupus), nephrotic syndrome, pregnancy or postpartum within 1 month, immobility, acquired or genetic thrombophilia, chronic lung disease.

- Contraindications to pharmacologic prophylaxis: heparin-induced thrombocytopenia, active bleeding, preoperative within 12 hours or postoperative within 24 hours, LP or epidural within 24 hours; recent intraocular or intracranial surgery; coagulopathy.

- Recommended regimens (for medical patients):

  - Low molecular weight heparins (LMWH): enoxaparin 40 mg sub-cutaneous q day or dalteparin 5,000 units subcutanous q day or fondaparinux 2.5 mg subcutaneous q day. Adjust dosage for CrCl <30 mg/dL.

  - Unfractionated heparin (UFH) 5,000 subcutaneous bid or tid.

  - For patients at high risk of bleeding, consider intermittent pneu-matic compression or graduated compression stockings.

- For planned invasive procedures (e.g., pacemaker placement, cathe-terization, surgery, etc.), hold UFH 8 hours prior to procedure and LMWH 12 hours prior to procedure!

GI PROPHYLAXIS

- Gastric erosions and stress-induced ulcers can form in critically ill patients. However, not every patient needs GI prophylaxis—if pa-tients do not have any of the risk factors listed below, prophylaxis is not necessary, even in the ICU setting! Most patient will *not* need GI prophylaxis.

- Risk factors for stress-induced ulcers: Mechanical ventilation >48 hours, coagulopathy, shock, sepsis, multi-organ system failure, he-patic failure, multiple trauma, burns >35% of total body surface area, organ transplant recipient, head trauma, spinal cord injury, history of peptic ulcer disease or upper GI bleeding, use of anticoagulants or high dose corticosteroids.

- Recommended regimens:

  - H_2 blockers: famotidine 20 mg PO/IV bid or ranitidine 50 mg PO/IV tid.

  - Proton-pump inhibitors: omeprazole 40 mg PO q day.

ASSESSMENT/PLAN

This is the meat of your note. It is useful to separate this section by problem. The assessment should include a one-line summary of the patient's known medical problems (i.e., HTN, T2DM, CAD) and those under evaluation (i.e., fever, melena). For example, 60 y/o female with a history of hypertension, T2DM presents with new onset chest pain. Include a short differential diagnosis of the current problem.

The plan should be separated by problem. Cover all problems, in-cluding stable issues:

1. Chest pain: No ECG changes, chest pain free now, will rule out MI, monitor on telemetry, continue beta blocker, nitrates, ASA, and ACE-I. NPO for stress thallium in AM assuming rules out for MI.

2. Hypertension: Good control on current medical regimen.

3. T2DM: Good control with A1C of 6.5. Continue glucose checks, prudent diabetic diet. Hold PO diabetic meds while NPO. Will use insulin sliding scale while NPO.

4. Fluids/electrolytes/nutrition (F/E/N): Monitor I/O's, urine output.

5. Vascular access: Note patient's sites of IV access.

6. Disposition: Note any discharge needs (nursing home placement, home health, home O_2, etc).

7. Code status: Code status should be addressed with every patient admitted regardless of age or disease. Unexpected problems arise too often, and it is better to be prepared.

LABORATORY RESULTS AND ORDERS

It is imperative that orders and lab tests are followed up in a timely manner. You must take personal responsibility to ensure that this is completed.

PATIENT SAFETY ISSUES
Restraints

Restraints may be needed for patients in a variety of situations. Indications for restraints include:

- Protecting patients from harming themselves (e.g., self-extubation, pulling at Foley catheter, pulling at IV lines).
- Protecting staff and/or family from patient violence.
- Facilitating medically necessary procedures.
- Preventing disoriented patients from wandering or falls.

Written orders for restraints must include:

- Type of restraint (e.g., Posey vest, soft limb restraints, mittens).
- Start and end times.
- Frequency of monitoring and re-evaluation.

Medical reason for restraint use must be documented in the chart. Patients should be re-evaluated at least every 24 hours and orders renewed if necessary. Consider the use of chemical restraints (e.g., benzodiazepines or antipsychotics), bedside sitters, bed alarms, or veil beds instead of physical restraints if possible. Most hospitals have written policies regarding the use of restraints—be sure your orders and documentation comply with hospital policies.

Dangerous Abbreviations For Order Writing

Each hospital may have its own list of unacceptable or dangerous abbreviations, but the table below shows some of the most common.

ABBREVIATION	INTENDED MEANING	MISINTER- PRETATION	CORRECTION
1.0 mg (zero after decimal point)	1 mg	Misread as 10 mg if decimal point not seen	Do not write zero by itself after a decimal point (X mg)
0.5 mg (no zero before decimal point)	0.5 mg	Misread as 5 mg	Always use a zero before a decimal point (0.X mg)
U or u	Units	Can be misread as an extra zero or four	Write out "unit"
IU	International units	Can be misread as IV or 10	Use "units"
µg	Microgram	Can be mistaken for milligrams	Use "mcg"
cc	Cubic centimeters	Misread as "U"	Use "mL"
qd, QD, qod, QOD	Every day or every other day	Mistaken as "qid"	Use "daily" or "every other day"

Abbreviation	Intended Meaning	Misinterpretation	Correction
x#d	e.g. q3d for 3 days or doses	Not clear if 3 days or 3 doses	Use "3 days" or "3 doses"
T.I.W.	Three times a week	Mistaken as "three times a day or twice weekly"	Write "three times weekly," specify dates to be given
MSO_4, MS, $MgSO_4$	Morphine sulfate or magnesium sulfate	Mistaken for each other	Write out drug names
per os	Orally	"os" can be mistaken for "right eye"	Use "PO," "by mouth," or "orally"
qhs	Nightly or at bedtime	Misinterpreted as every hour	Use "nightly" or "at bedtime"
q6 PM, etc.	Every evening at 6	Misread as every 6 hours	Use "6 PM nightly"
AU, AS, AD	Both ears, right ear, left ear	Misinterpreted as OU (both eyes), OS (left eye), OD (right eye)	Do not use, write out specific directions
SC or SQ	Subcutaneous	Mistaken as "SL" when poorly written	Write "subcut." or "subcutaneous"

9   Daily Assessments

... Same bat time, same bat channel ...

ROUNDS

... Round and round and round ...

Many programs categorize rounds into prerounds, work rounds, and attending rounds.

Prerounding

Prerounding is primarily an intern's responsibility. Usually allow 30 minutes to an hour before rounds, depending on the number of patients on your service. The exact responsibilities should be worked out individually with your resident. It is often not necessary to physically see all of your patients before work rounds. It is customary to see those patients with an acute problem.

Probably the most important aspects are getting signouts and catching up on the overnight events (i.e., cross-cover problems). However, the following example is a good prerounding plan:

1. Get your signout from the night float or cross-cover team. You need to know of any major events that happened overnight, and this dictates how you will spend your time prerounding.

2. Check vital signs on all your patients. This can often be done on the computers. It is also helpful to check nursing notes on the computer.

3. See the patients. A quick check on your patients (2–3 minutes per patient) allows you to see how they look and if they have developed any new problems overnight. Of course, patients with more acute illness require more time.

4. Check lab results and final results of tests (i.e., CXR, Echos, etc.). Check telemetry every day on all your monitored patients.

5. For patients with private physicians, it is often helpful to discuss the plan face to face with them in the morning (i.e., try to catch them on their morning rounds). This saves you time in trying to reach them at their offices or in deciphering their progress notes.

DAILY NOTES AND EVALUATION

Interns are primarily responsible for writing daily notes on each of their patients. The SOAP format is usually used for daily notes.

Subjective: What the patient says or what nursing staff reports. Past 24 hour events.

Objective: Factual information, vitals, PE, lab results, lines, and tubes. Include microbiology results, x-rays, and other studies here. Always check final official readings of tests.

Assessment/Plan: This is the meat of the note. Usually categorized by problem or organ system in the order of importance. Always include fluids/electrolytes/nutrition as a problem as well as code status in every note. Also include the type of IV access the patient has. In addition, the last category or problem should be discharge planning. Include status and goals (e.g., social work placement, home oxygen).

Active medications are often listed in a side column. This exercise can be tedious but ensures that every medication is reviewed daily. Also include the day number for antibiotics and other loading dose medications.

Review the following items daily:

- Do IV lines need to be changed?
- Can IV meds be changed to PO?
- Can you discontinue the Foley?
- Do restraint orders need to be renewed?
- Can you advance the diet and increase the activity of the patient? Is the patient moving his or her bowels? Is there any procedure or test planned that requires that patient to be NPO?
- PT/OT and social work: Are they involved, and should they be? What is the status of discharge planning?
- Are all meds adjusted for renal or hepatic failure?

Daily orders should be consolidated and written as early as possible. Don't forget to order AM labs for the next morning. Every lab test and study ordered needs to be followed up. If a study needs to be done stat or ASAP, you must notify the ward clerk and nurse directly, and consider talking to the radiologist directly. It is often helpful to discuss a brief plan with the patient and the nursing staff. This helps them to be part of the team and also helps move things along.

DISCHARGE PLANNING

D/C planning must be addressed and readdressed constantly. Proper D/C planning prevents large teams and reduces resident irritation. D/C planning should start on admission. Social work should be consulted on admission if D/C needs are anticipated (assisted living, placement, transportation). Scheduled meetings with case coordinators or social workers are often helpful to reassess the situation and provide updates.

SIGNOUTS

Most programs have some variety of night float to help with cross-cover overnight. Succinct but complete signouts include the following items:

- Name of patient, birth date, room number.

- List of active problems and relevant medical history (i.e., ESRD).

- Any pending studies or overnight lab tests and trends of lab results. Also include certain criteria to act on (i.e., transfuse 1 unit PRBC if Hct is <28).

- Code status: This must be specified.

- Highlight any worrisome patients and why you are concerned. Include suggestions on how to deal with certain problems and what worked earlier in the hospital course.

10 Other Notes of Importance

... The paper chase ...

OFF-SERVICE NOTES

... Passing the buck ...

It is your final day on the floors, you've had a grueling month, and the last thing you want to do is write another note, let alone think about writing long, drawn-out off-service notes. However, the presence of short concise off-service notes can be a life-saver to the intern coming onto the service. The essentials include the following items:

1. Date of admission.

2. Major diagnoses.

3. Pertinent past medical history.

4. Hospital course (major interventions, events, procedures); this can be organized chronologically or by organ system depending on the patient.

5. Current medications including day number for antibiotics.

6. Current pertinent PE and lab results.

7. Assessment and plan.

PROCEDURE NOTES

... See one, do one, document one ...

These are of vital importance as part of the documentation of the hospital course and should include the following items:

1. Procedure, site of procedure.

2. Indication(s).

3. Consent.

4. Sterile prep used.

5. Anesthesia used.

6. Brief description of the procedure.

7. Specimens and what they were sent for.

8. Complications.

9. Postprocedure disposition and pending follow-up studies (i.e., CXR post–central line placement).

10. Any fluids that you just spent your valuable time collecting should be hand delivered to the lab personally (e.g., CSF, ABG, other taps, etc.).

DEATH/EXPIRATIONS

... The celestial discharge ...

Interns are called on quite frequently to pronounce a death. Certain steps must be performed.

- On arrival to the bedside, you should observe for respirations, auscultate for heart sounds, palpate for a pulse, and attempt to elicit a corneal reflex. You also need to agree on an exact time of death with the nursing staff.

- Notify the private physician and family immediately, even in the middle of the night. The family must be asked specifically about (1) autopsy, (2) anatomic gift donation, and (3) funeral home. Appropriate forms for an autopsy and anatomic gifts must be completed. **Note:** Many hospitals have specially trained personnel to handle these particular requests, so be aware that it may not be appropriate for you to approach the family regarding these issues. Notify the appropriate hospital personnel if necessary.

- Complete a death note in the progress note section of the chart. It should include the following information: ''Called by nursing to see patient regarding unresponsiveness. The patient was found to be breathless, pulseless, and without heart tones, blood pressure, and corneal reflexes. The patient was pronounced dead at 5:25 AM on April 29th, 2005. The patient's private physician and family were notified. The patient's family refused both anatomic gifts and autopsy. The funeral home will be Manchester Mortuary.'' The word *dead* must be used.

- The Certificate of Death must be completed. If the patient has a private physician, the death certificate will be completed by the private physician. Also, dictate a short death summary at this time.

11   Discharges

... Happy Trails! Come back if you have to ...

With proper planning, discharges can be smooth for you and the patient. In today's environment, many more diseases are being managed and followed in the outpatient setting. Therefore, it is critical that the patient has follow-up and the patient's physician is aware of any pending issues or studies. Communication with all involved parties is crucial to a successful discharge process. It also prevents many bounce backs.

DISCHARGE PROCESS/PEARLS

- Obtain social work/case coordinator assistance early in the admission. Try to anticipate issues and problems early on (e.g., transportation, home oxygen, or placement).

- Make sure the patient and his or her family are aware of possible discharge dates so they can arrange their schedules and not be caught off guard.

- Arrange for home services at least 1 day before discharge (i.e., home nursing, PT, OT, etc.).

- Criteria for home O_2:

    PaO_2 <55 mm Hg
    PaO_2 of 55–59 mm Hg with evidence of cor pulmonale or secondary polycythemia (Hct >55%)
    O_2 sat <88% on room air consistently (at rest, with exercise, or with sleep)

- Get rid of Foley catheters, telemetry monitoring, and supplemental oxygen as soon as possible. Many rehabilitation facilities require that these are not present 24 hours before discharge.

- Change antibiotics to PO the day before discharge. Avoid AM lab work the morning of discharge, unless absolutely necessary.

- Provide all prescription medications including three refills, excluding controlled substances. This paperwork can often be done in advance.

- Dictate the discharge summary at the time of discharge. It may seem painful at the time, but it will save you time later. It is most efficient to dictate when you are most familiar with the patient and hospital course. Take the extra 5–10 minutes to complete it now.

- The hospital course section of a well-organized discharge summary is generally organized by problem list.

DISCHARGE SUMMARY

Each institution has its own rules on discharge summaries. However, most should include the following items:

- Your name, the attending physician's name, and patient name and number.
- Date of admission and discharge.
- Principal and secondary diagnoses and procedures.
- Chief complaint and HPI.
- Hospital course, including all major events, listing of major radiological and diagnostic test and results, and all major therapeutic interventions.
- Discharge medications, diet, and activity.
- Follow-up plans.
- Condition on discharge.
- Copy distribution.

12 Top Ten Workups

CHEST PAIN

... You may start to develop chest pain of your own ...

Of course, angina or MI is your first thought. However, the most important tool in identifying the cause of chest pain is a good history. The patient should be assessed immediately.

Before you hang up the phone, ask the nurse for vital signs. Initial verbal orders should include stat ECG; O_2 by NC to keep saturations >92%; sublingual nitroglycerin 0.4 mg and aspirin 325 mg to bedside. Confirm IV access.

Major Causes of Chest Pain

Heart/vascular: Angina, MI, acute pericarditis, aortic dissection.
Lungs: Pneumonia, PE, pneumothorax.
GI: Esophageal spasm, GERD, PUD, pancreatitis.
Other: Costochondritis, herpes zoster.

Things You Don't Want to Miss (Call Your Resident)

MI
Aortic dissection
PE
Pneumothorax

Key History

- Check BP, pulse, respirations, and O_2 saturations.
- Quickly review chart.
- Take a focused history including quality, duration, radiation, changes with respiration, diaphoresis, and N/V.
- Review ECG. If cardiac etiology is suspected, give NTG SL if SBP >90. Also, make patient chew the aspirin, if not already given during the day.

Focused Examination

	KEY POINTS
General	How distressed or sick does the patient look?
Vitals	Hypotension is an ominous sign. Tachycardia may be from a PE or from pain. Bradycardia may be from AV block with inferior MI. Take BP in both arms.

KEY POINTS

Chest	Check for chest wall tenderness and any skin lesions. Listen for murmur, rubs, or gallops. Assess JVP.
Lungs	Assess for crackles, absent breath sounds on one side, friction rub.
Abdomen	Tenderness, bowel sounds.
Extremities	Edema or evidence of deep venous thrombosis. If dissection is suspected, examine pulses bilaterally in both upper and lower extremities.

Laboratory Data

Obtain an ECG if you haven't already. Check ABG if respiratory distress or low saturations are present; serial troponins (q12h × 2), portable CXR. Consider V/Q scan or spiral CT scan if PE is suspected; also consider lower extremity Dopplers or D-dimer. Consider contrast CT or TEE if dissection is suspected.

Management

- Cardiac: If evidence of acute MI on ECG (ST elevation of 1 mm or more in two contiguous leads or new LBBB) and history, call a stat cardiology consult for consideration of reperfusion therapy (thrombolytics or angioplasty). Ensure the patient is on a monitor, has IV access, has oxygen 2 L by NC, and has received an aspirin. Consider administering β-blockers, nitrates, morphine, heparin (UFH or LMWH). Metoprolol, 5 mg IV, may be initiated and repeated every 5 minutes for a total dose of 15 mg.

- Angina: NTG, 0.4 mg times 3 every 5 minutes, assuming SBP >90. Consider β-blockers, nitrates, heparin, and antiplatelet agents. Place on telemetry. If patient is still having chest pain after SLNTG × 3, consider giving morphine and starting NTG drip, titrate until chest pain free.

- Aortic dissection: Arrange for immediate transfer to CCU/MICU. Start nitroprusside or labetalol for BP control. Stat vascular/thoracic surgery consult.

- Pulmonary: If PE, ensure adequate oxygenation and administer IV heparin or LMWH. See Therapeutics section for dosing (Chap. 15).

- Pneumothorax: Tension pneumothorax requires immediate needle decompression in the second intercostal space in the midclavicular line, followed by chest tube. Other pneumothoraces involving >20% of the lung require a surgery consult for chest tube placement.

- GI: Antacids such as aluminum hydroxide (Maalox), 30 mL PO prn q4–6h (avoid in patients with renal failure), famotidine (Pepcid), 20 mg PO bid, or omeprazole (Prilosec), 20 mg PO q day. Elevate the head of the bed.

Refractory Chest Pain

- Re-evaluate patient for causes of chest pain—has your initial impression changed?

- Repeat ECG, vital signs, physical exam.

- For ongoing cardiac ischemia, particularly with elevated troponins and/or ST segment depression, start a NTG drip, consider adding a glycoprotein IIb/IIIa inhibitor (e.g., eptifibatide or tirofiban), and consider an urgent cardiology consult.

ABDOMINAL PAIN

… Not just from the cafeteria food …

What are the patient's vital signs? How severe is the pain? Is this a new problem? If vital signs are stable, inform the nurse you will be there shortly and to call you immediately if things worsen before you arrive.

Major Causes of Abdominal Pain (See Figure 12-1)

It's easiest to think of them by location:

Right upper quadrant

L, Liver (hepatitis, abscess, perihepatitis)
GB, Gallbladder (cholecystitis, cholangitis, choledocholithiasis)
HF, Hepatic flexure (obstruction)

Right lower quadrant

A, Appendix (appendicitis,* abscess)
O, Ovary (torsion, ruptured cyst, carcinoma)

Left upper quadrant

Sp, Spleen (rupture, infarct, abscess)
SF, Splenic flexure (obstruction)

Left lower quadrant

LC, Left colon (diverticulitis, ischemic colitis)
O, Ovary (torsion, ruptured cyst, carcinoma)

Epigastrium

> H, Heart (myocardial infarction, pericarditis, aortic dissection)
> AAA, Abdominal aortic aneurysm
> Lu, Lung (pneumonia, pleurisy)
> SA, Subphrenic abscess
> E, Esophagus (gastroesophageal reflux disease)
> S, Stomach and duodenum (peptic ulcer)
> P, Pancreas (pancreatitis)
> K, Kidney (pyelonephritis, renal colic)

Hypogastrium

> K, Kidney (renal colic)
> PA, Psoas abscess
> I, Intestine (infection,* obstruction,* inflammatory bowel disease*)
> O, Ovary (torsion, ruptured cyst, carcinoma)
> OT, Ovarian tube (ectopic pregnancy, salpingitis, endometriosis)
> B, Bladder (cystitis, distended bladder)

Generalized abdominal pain

> 1. See conditions marked with an asterisk (*)
>
> 2. Peritonitis (any cause)
>
> 3. Diabetic ketoacidosis
>
> 4. Sickle cell crisis
>
> 5. Acute intermittent porphyria
>
> 6. Acute adrenocortical insufficiency due to steroid withdrawal

From Marshall SA, Ruedy J. *On call: principles and protocols,* 3rd ed. Philadelphia: W.B. Saunders Company, 2000.

Things You Don't Want to Miss (Call Your Resident)

AAA rupture
Bowel rupture, perforation, or ischemia
Ascending cholangitis
Acute appendicitis
Retroperitoneal hematoma

Key History

- Check BP, pulse, respirations, O_2 saturations, and temperature.

- Quickly look at the patient and review the chart.

- Take a focused history, including quality, duration, radiation, changes with respiration, location, N/V (bilious versus nonbilious),

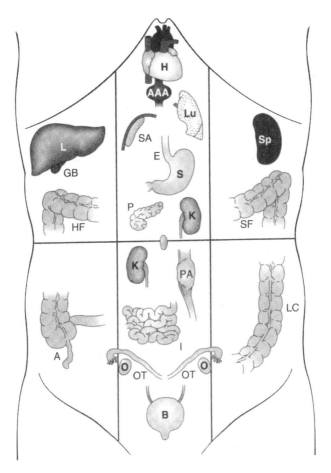

FIGURE 12-1 Major causes of abdominal pain.

last bowel movement, and any hematemesis or melena or hemato-chezia. For women of childbearing age, ask about their last menstrual period.

- Mesenteric ischemia often has pain out of proportion to examination. Consider this, especially with a history of atrial fibrillation, vascular disease, and in elderly patients.

Focused Examination

	KEY POINTS
General	How distressed or sick does the patient look?
Vitals	Repeat now.
HEENT	Check for icterus.
Chest	Check for any skin lesions. Listen for murmur, rubs, or gallops. Assess jugular venous pulse.
Lungs	Assess for crackles, absent breath sounds on one side, friction rub.
Abdomen	Inspect bowel sounds: high pitched with SBO, absent with ileus. Percussion: tympany, shifting dullness. Palpation: guarding, rebound tenderness, Murphy's sign, psoas, and obturator signs. Assess for CVA tenderness.
Rectal	Must be performed, guaiac for occult blood.
Pelvic	If indicated by history.

Laboratory Data

Consider CBC, electrolytes, ABG, lactate, LFTs, amylase, lipase, β- hCG, and UA. Films to consider include flat and upright abdominal films, CXR, and ECG. Abdominal CT, ultrasound, or both may be required.

Management

- The initial goal is to determine if the patient has an acute abdomen and needs surgical evaluation and treatment. Avoid any analgesics as this may mask the pain and obscure the evaluation. An acute abdomen includes such signs as rebound tenderness or guarding and conditions such as ruptured viscus, abscess, or hemorrhage. See Acute Abdomen section in the General Surgery consult section (Chap. 17).

- Other conditions can be managed using a more detailed and leisurely approach, after the acute abdomen has been ruled out.

- Keep the patient NPO. Ensure IV access and run maintenance fluids.

ACUTE ALTERED MENTAL STATUS

... Not unlike you postcall ...

What are the patient's vital signs? What was the time course of changes? Any change in level of consciousness or any trauma? Is the patient a diabetic? Any recent narcotics or sedatives given? What was the reason for admission (e.g., alcohol or drug intoxication/withdrawal)?

Initial verbal orders to consider: think of TONG (thiamine, oxygen, naloxone, and glucose). Have the nurse obtain Accucheck and oxygen saturations now.

Acute mental status changes associated with fever or decreased consciousness require that you see the patient immediately.

Major Causes of Acute Altered Mental Status

- Structural/CNS

  Head trauma/subdural hematoma
  Hydrocephalus
  CVA/TIA
  Dementia
  Postictal state
  Fecal impaction
  Tumor or abscess

- Systemic/metabolic

  Drugs (narcotics, benzos, anticholinergics, psychoactive medications, etc.), especially in elderly, even in low doses
  Alcohol withdrawal
  Hypoglycemia/DKA
  Organ failure (hypoxia, hypercapnia, uremia, or hepatic encephalopathy)
  Hypertension or hypotension
  Infection (sepsis, UTI, meningitis), especially in the setting of dementia
  Endocrine (thyroid disease, Addison's disease, hypercalcemia, B_{12} deficiency)

Things You Don't Want to Miss (Call Your Resident)

Sepsis or meningitis
Intracranial mass or increased pressure
Alcohol withdrawal (DTs)
Acute CVA

Key History

- Check BP, pulse, respirations, O_2 saturations, temperature, and Accucheck.

- Quickly look at the patient and review the chart.
- Confirm no falls or trauma.
- Review chart for new meds or narcotics.
- Take a focused history, including onset and level of responsiveness.

Focused Examination

	KEY POINTS
General	How distressed or sick does the patient look?
HEENT	Look for signs of trauma; pupil size, symmetry, and response to light; papilledema and nuchal rigidity.
Abdomen	Look for ascites, jaundice, and other signs of liver disease.
Neurologic	Thoroughly examine, including mental status examination, and check for asterixis.

Laboratory Data

Consider CBC, electrolytes, LFTs, ABG, TSH, ammonia level, UA, cultures, ECG, and CXR. Other studies that may be required are lumbar puncture, CT, and EEG. Never perform a lumbar puncture if you suspect a mass lesion or raised intracranial pressure until a CT is obtained or a funduscopic examination is performed.

Management

- Management is based on findings on examination and laboratory data. If meningitis is suspected, lumbar puncture should be performed after CT or funduscopic examination. In addition, empiric antibiotics should be started stat (see Chap. 17, Neurology consult section, for antibiotic choices).

- Alcohol withdrawal needs to be treated urgently with benzodiazepines, usually with chlordiazepoxide (Librium) 100 mg PO tid or lorazepam (Ativan) 0.5–1 mg PO/IV/IM q6–8h (prn or scheduled). Thiamine should also be administered, especially before any glucose. See Chapter 13 for further management strategies.

ACUTE RENAL FAILURE

… Like you have time to use the bathroom …

What are the patient's vital signs? How much urine has been produced in the last 24 hours? In the last 8 hours? Does the patient have a Foley catheter inserted? What are the patient's recent electrolytes, especially potassium, BUN, creatinine, and bicarbonate?

If the patient does have a Foley catheter inserted, ask the nurse to flush the catheter with 30 mL NS. If the patient does not have a Foley catheter, ask the nurse to place one now. Tell the nurse you will see the patient shortly.

Major Causes of Oliguria

Oliguria is generally defined as <400 mL of urine per 24 hours. Major causes of oliguria can be broken down as follows:

- Prerenal: Volume depletion, congestive heart failure, vascular occlusion

- Renal: Glomerular, tubular/interstitial (acute tubular necrosis caused by drugs or toxins), and vascular

- Postrenal: Obstruction (BPH), clogged Foley catheter, stones

Things You Don't Want to Miss (Call Your Resident)

Hyperkalemia

Key History

- Check BP, pulse, respirations, O_2 saturations, and temperature.

- Quickly look at the patient and review the chart.

- Take a focused history.

- Determining volume status is important. Review ins and outs over the past few days. Any new medications (e.g., ACE inhibitors, diuretics, NSAIDs, IV contrast dye)?

Focused Examination

	KEY POINTS
General	How distressed or sick does the patient look?
Vitals	Check orthostatics and weight over the past few days.
Cardiovascular	Check for JVD, friction rub, and skin turgor.
Abdomen	Look for ascites or enlarged bladder.
Genitourinary	Check for enlarged prostate.
Extremities	Assess perfusion. Check for asterixis.

Laboratory Data

UA: Look for cells, casts, protein. Consider electrolytes, urine electrolytes, calculate FENa (or FEurea), urine eosinophils, ABG, and ECG. Renal ultrasound should be ordered within 24 hours to rule out hydronephrosis and evaluate the renal system.

Management

- The minimum acceptable urine output is 30 mL/hour. If flushing the Foley catheter did not help, ask the nurse to change the Foley catheter.

- Initial management should be directed at treating life-threatening electrolyte disorders and correcting volume contraction and hypotension. Obtain diagnostic urinary studies before administering diuretics. Don't forget to adjust drug doses based on glomerular filtration rate.

- Calculate the fractional excretion of sodium:

$$FENa = \frac{U[Na] \times P[Cr]}{U[Cr] \times P[Na]}$$

  This equation is most useful with oliguric renal failure but may be helpful in nonoliguric renal failure. FENa >1% to 2% with oliguria is almost always ATN but can be prerenal with diuretics. FENa <1% with oliguria is generally prerenal: volume depletion, severe CHF, or nephrotic syndrome, NSAID or dye toxicity, sepsis, cyclosporine toxicity, acute GN, and hepatorenal syndrome. Can calculate FEurea in nonoliguric renal failure or if diuretics have been given. FEurea <35% is consistent with prerenal state.

- Hyperkalemia, CHF, severe acidemia, and pericarditis require immediate attention. Obtain recent electrolytes and a stat potassium.

- If hyperkalemia suspected, order an ECG. A stat renal consult is required if the patient needs urgent dialysis. Indications for urgent dialysis include

  1. Hyperkalemia (unable to reduce medically)
  2. Volume overload
  3. Acidemia pH <7.2
  4. Uremic encephalopathy
  5. Uremic pericarditis

  Treatment of hyperkalemia is covered in Chapter 13.

- **Prerenal causes** can be initially managed with a small volume challenge, such as 250–500 mL NS bolus depending on the cardiovascular status of the patient. This can be followed by NS at a set rate. Specific criteria should be given to the nursing staff (i.e., call HO if urine output is <30 mL/hr). Alternatively, if congestive heart failure is suspected, the patient may need diuresis. Escalating doses of furosemide (Lasix) can be used, and urine output and daily weights can be assessed. With a fluid challenge, the creatinine level often trends down by the next morning if the cause is prerenal.

- **Postrenal causes** can be potentially managed by placing a Foley catheter. If immediate flow is obtained, urethral obstruction is likely. If a Foley cannot be placed due to obstruction, consider a urology consultation.

- For **contrast-induced ARF prophylaxis**, normovolemia is essential. Use $^1/_2$ NS or NS at 1 mg/kg/hr for 6–12 hours before and 6–12 hours after the procedure.

HEADACHE

... Like your head isn't pounding by now ...

What are the patient's vital signs? How severe is the headache? Has there been a change in consciousness? Has the patient had similar headaches in the past; if so, what relieves them?

If the headache is severe and acute or associated with N/V, changes in vision, fever, or decreased consciousness, the patient should be seen immediately. Otherwise, inform the nurse you will see the patient shortly.

Major Causes of Headache

Tension
Vascular (migraine, subarachnoid hemorrhage)
Cluster
Drugs
Temporal arteritis
Infectious (meningitis, sinusitis)
Trauma
CVA
Hypertension
Mass lesions

Things You Don't Want to Miss (Call Your Resident)

Meningitis
Subarachnoid hemorrhage or subdural hematoma
Mass lesion associated with herniation

Key History

- Check BP, pulse, respirations, O_2 saturations, and temperature.

- Quickly look at the patient and review the chart.

- A detailed, well-focused history is the best method for evaluating a headache. Most are tension or migraine type, but more serious conditions need to be ruled out.

Focused Examination

	KEY POINTS
General	How distressed or sick does the patient look?
HEENT	Look for signs of trauma, pupil size, symmetry, response to light, papilledema, nuchal rigidity, temporal artery tenderness, and sinus tenderness.
Neurologic	Thorough examination, including mental status.

Laboratory Data

Consider CBC and ESR if temporal arteritis suspected. Head CT should be considered for:

1. A chronic headache pattern that has changed or a new severe headache occurs.

2. A new headache in a patient older than 50 years.

3. Focal findings on neurologic examination.

If meningitis is suspected, lumbar puncture should be performed. If there is no papilledema and no focal neurologic findings, lumbar puncture should not be delayed for a CT scan, especially if the CT cannot be done within 1 hour.

Management

- The initial goal is to exclude the serious life-threatening conditions mentioned previously. After such conditions have been excluded, management can focus on symptomatic relief.

- For suspected bacterial meningitis, start antibiotics immediately. See Chapter 17, Neurology consult section, for antibiotic choices.

- For suspected subdural hematoma or subarachnoid hemorrhage, obtain CT scan. If positive, a neurosurgery consultation should be obtained.

- Tension headaches and mild migraines can be treated with acetaminophen (Tylenol), 650–1,000 mg PO q6h prn or ibuprofen (Motrin), 200–600 mg PO q6–8h, consider sumatriptan (Imitrex), 25 mg PO for moderate to severe migraine headaches; can repeat 25–100 mg q2h for maximum of 200–300 mg/day.

- Severe migraines may require a narcotic such as meperidine or codeine. Sumatriptan or ergotamine are usually most effective in the prodromal stage. These agents are contraindicated in patients with angina, uncontrolled hypertension, hemiplegia, or basilar artery migraine.

HYPOTENSION AND HYPERTENSION

... Too high, too low, uh oh ...

Hypotension

What are the patient's vital signs? Is the patient conscious, confused, or disoriented? What has the patient's blood pressure been? What was the reason for admission?

If impending or established shock is suspected, ensure IV access (at least 20 gauge IV) and have the patient placed in Trendelenburg's position (head of bed down). Hypotension requires that you see the patient immediately.

Major Causes of Hypotension

Cardiogenic (rate or pump problem)
Hypovolemic
Septic shock
Anaphylaxis

Things You Don't Want to Miss (Call Your Resident)

Shock, which is evidence of inadequate perfusion. This is best assessed by looking at end organs: brain (mental status), heart (chest pain), kidneys (urine output), and skin (cool, clammy). Shock is a clinical diagnosis defined as a systolic BP <90, with evidence of inadequate tissue perfusion.

Key History

- Check BP (both arms), pulse, respirations, O_2 saturations, and temperature.

- Quickly look at the patient and review chart. Get an ECG.

Focused Examination

	KEY POINTS
General	How distressed or sick does the patient look?
Vitals	Repeat now. Elevated temperature and hypotension suggest sepsis.
Neurologic	Mentation.

	KEY POINTS
Cardiovascular	Heart rate, JVP, skin temperature, and color. Capillary refill.
Lungs	Listen for crackles, breath sounds on both sides.
GI	Any evidence of blood loss?

Laboratory Data

Consider troponins, ECG, ABG, CBC, electrolytes, and CXR.

Management

- Examine the ECG and take the pulse yourself. Check BP in both arms. A compensatory sinus tachycardia is an expected appropriate response to hypotension. However, check the ECG to ensure that the patient does not have atrial fibrillation, SVT, or ventricular tachycardia, which may cause hypotension because of decreased diastolic filling. Bradycardia may be seen in autonomic dysfunction or heart block.

- Most causes of shock require fluids to normalize the intravascular volume. Use normal saline or lactated Ringer's. The exception is cardiogenic shock, which may require preload and afterload reduction, inotropic and/or vasopressor support, and transfer to an ICU.

- Hypovolemic, anaphylactic, and septic shock require fluids. Use boluses of 500 mL to 1 L. If no response, repeat bolus or leave fluids open.

- Anaphylactic shock requires epinephrine, 0.3 mg IV immediately and repeated every 10–15 minutes as required. Hydrocortisone, 500 mg IV, and diphenhydramine (Benadryl), 25 mg IV, should also be administered.

- In septic shock, IV fluids and antibiotics can resolve the shock. However, continuing hypotension requires ICU admission for vasopressors.

- Cardiogenic shock can be the result of an acute MI or worsening CHF. However, other causes of hypotension and elevated JVP include acute cardiac tamponade, PE, and tension pneumothorax. These always need to be considered.

Hypertension

... Feel YOUR blood pressure rising? ...

What are the patient's vital signs? What has the patient's blood pressure been? What is the reason for admission? What BP medications has the patient been taking? Does the patient have signs of hypertensive emergency?

The rate of rise of the BP and the setting in which the high BP is occurring are more important than the level of BP itself. Elevated blood pressure alone, in the absence of symptoms or new or progressive target organ damage, rarely requires emergent therapy.

Hypertensive emergencies require that you see the patient immediately. Make sure the patient has an IV and order an ECG. Inform the nurse that you will arrive shortly.

Hypertensive Emergencies

Encephalopathy
Intracranial hemorrhage
Unstable angina or MI
Acute left ventricular failure with pulmonary edema
Aortic dissection
Eclampsia
Renal insufficiency (new or worsened)

Hypertensive Urgencies

Blood pressure >180/110
Optic disc edema
Severe perioperative hypertension

Things You Don't Want to Miss (*Call Your Resident*)

Hypertensive emergencies

Key History

- Check BP, pulse, respirations, O_2 saturations, and temperature.

- Quickly look at the patient and review the chart. Get an ECG.

Focused Examination

	KEY POINTS
General	How distressed or sick does the patient look?
Vitals	Repeat BP now in both arms.
Neurologic	Mentation, confusion, delirium, focal neurologic deficits.

KEY POINTS

HEENT	Fundi for papilledema, retinal hemorrhages, or hypertensive changes.
Cardiovascular	Heart rate, jugular venous pulse, color. Capillary refill.
Lungs	Listen for crackles, breath sounds on both sides.

Laboratory Data

Consider troponins, ECG, ABG, CBC, electrolytes, UA, and CXR.

Management

- Treat the patient, not the BP reading. Acute lowering of BP of asymptomatic patients with long-standing hypertension can be dangerous.

- Hypertensive emergencies require an ICU setting. Goal is to reduce the MAP by no more than 25% in the first 2 hours. IV hydralazine, nitroprusside, labetalol, or enalaprilat are often used. While arranging transfer to the ICU, certain wards allow medications to be started. Consider IV nitroglycerin for hypertension associated with MI or pulmonary edema. Nitroprusside and labetolol are useful in aortic dissection. Nitroprusside is also used for patients with encephalopathy but often requires intra-arterial blood pressure monitoring.

- Hypertensive urgencies can usually be managed with oral medications with the goal of reducing BP over 24–48 hours. Examples include captopril, 25 mg PO, clonidine, 0.1 mg PO, or labetalol, 200–400 mg PO. These can be repeated or titrated every 2–4 hours. Close follow-up is essential.

COMMON ARRHYTHMIAS

... Too fast, too slow, or too irregular ...

What are the patient's vital signs, including temperature? Any chest pain or shortness of breath?

Order a stat ECG. Patients with chest pain, shortness of breath, or hypotension need to be seen immediately.

Major Causes of Rapid Heart Rate and Slow Rates

- Rapid rates

  Regular: sinus tachycardia, SVT, ventricular tachycardia, atrial flutter

  Irregular: atrial fibrillation, multifocal atrial tachycardia

- Slow rates

   Drugs (β-blockers, CCB, digoxin)
   Sick sinus syndrome
   MI (especially inferior)
   AV block

Things You Don't Want to Miss (Call Your Resident)

Ventricular tachycardia
Hypotension or angina or MI

Key History

- Check BP, pulse, respirations, O_2 saturations, and temperature.

- Quick look at patient and quick review of chart. Get an ECG.

Focused Examination

	KEY POINTS
General	How distressed or sick does the patient look?
Vitals	Repeat now.
Neurologic	Mentation.
Cardiovascular	Heart rate, jugular venous pulse, skin temperature and color, capillary refill.
Lungs	Listen for crackles and breath sounds on both sides.

Laboratory Data

Consider troponins, ECG, ABG, CBC, electrolytes, and CXR.

Management

- Always complete the ABCs first and ensure O_2, and IV access. Place patient on monitor or telemetry; consider transfer to a monitored bed on a cardiology floor.

- If patient is hypotensive and has atrial fibrillation with RVR, SVT, or ventricular tachycardia, emergency cardioversion may be required.

- In general, if the patient is unstable with serious signs or symptoms, a ventricular rate greater than 150, or both, you should prepare for immediate cardioversion. The patient may require sedation—call your resident. Serious signs and symptoms per ACLS protocol include chest pain, shortness of breath, decreased level of consciousness, hypotension and shock, congestive heart failure, and acute MI. Refer to the proper ACLS algorithm at this point (see Chap. 2) and call your resident.

- Atrial fibrillation with rapid rate but without evidence of hemodynamic compromise can be rate controlled with diltiazem, metoprolol, or digoxin. Amiodarone can also be considered. See ECG section (Chap. 16) for dosing.

- SVT without evidence of hemodynamic compromise can sometimes be broken with Valsalva's maneuver, carotid sinus massage (one side at a time and always listen for bruits first), or both. If still in SVT, try adenosine, 6 mg rapid IV push, followed by 12 mg rapid IV push if necessary. If the complex width is narrow with stable BP, verapamil, 2.5–5 mg IV, or diltiazem, 10 mg IV, can be used. If wide complex, manage as stable VT.

- For ventricular tachycardia, if pulseless or without BP, manage as ventricular fibrillation. If ventricular tachycardia with serious signs or symptoms, consider immediate synchronized cardioversion. If stable, follow the ACLS protocol (see Chap. 2).

FEVER

... Of known or unknown origin ...

What are the patient's vital signs? What was the reason for admission? Is this a new finding? Any associated symptoms (e.g., cough, headache, change in mental status, N/V, and so forth)? Any antipyretics or current antibiotics? Any recent surgeries (think of postoperative fever)?

Order blood and urine cultures. Patients with meningitis symptoms or hypotension need to be seen immediately.

Major Causes of Fever

- Infections: Best to think of by site—lung, urine, IV sites, blood, CNS, abdomen and pelvis, GI. Consider immune status.

- Drug-induced fever: Many drugs have been implicated.

- Atelectasis (especially post-op).

- Neoplasms.

- Connective tissue diseases.

- Deep venous thrombosis/pulmonary embolism.

- Fever of unknown origin.

Things You Don't Want To Miss

Meningitis
Septic shock

Key History

- Check BP, pulse, respirations, O_2 saturations, and temperature.

- Quickly look at the patient and review the chart.

Focused Examination

	KEY POINTS
General	How distressed or sick does the patient look? Check all catheter sites (IV, central line, Foley, G-tube, etc.)
Vitals	Repeat now. Tachycardia is an expected finding with fever. Recheck blood pressure.
Neurologic	Mentation, photophobia, neck stiffness, Brudzinski's or Kernig's signs.
Cardiovascular	Heart rate, jugular venous pulse, skin temperature and color. Any new murmurs? Capillary refill.
Lungs	Listen for crackles and breath sounds on both sides.
Abdomen	Assess for RUQ tenderness and bowel sounds.
Extremities	Check calves for signs of deep venous thrombosis, joints for effusions.

Laboratory Data

Consider CBC, blood cultures (two sets at different sites; if a central line is present, be sure to get one peripheral set as well), CMP, UA and culture, sputum culture and Gram's stain, CXR. LP if meningitis is suspected. Consider *Clostridium difficile* stool cultures.

Management

- Make sure the patient is hemodynamically stable. Review medications and obtain cultures. Give antipyretics (acetaminophen 650 mg PO/PR or ibuprofen 400 mg PO q 6–8 hours PRN). Ensure IV access and consider maintenance fluids including insensible losses.

- Consider antibiotics. If the patient is hemodynamically stable, immunocompetent, not toxic appearing, with no clear source of infection, it may be prudent to withhold antibiotics and recheck cultures.

- Patients with fever and hypotension require broad-spectrum antibiotics and IV fluids or pressors to manage the hypotension. Septic shock is an emergency. (Please refer to Hypotension Management earlier in this chapter.)

- Patients with fever and neutropenia (<500 cells/mm^3) require a careful physical examination, with particular attention paid to mucosal surfaces, lungs, skin, and vascular access sites. Blood cultures for bacteria and fungi should be drawn, also consider urine culture, sputum culture, LP, and CXR if clinically indicated. Broad spectrum antibiotics should be started. Choices for initial therapy include cefepime, ceftazidime, carbapenem or an antipseudomonal penicillin, with or without aminoglycoside. If a catheter-related infection is suspected or the patient is known to be colonized with penicillin-resistant pneumococcus or methicillin-resistant *S. aureus*, consider adding vancomycin to the above regimen.

- Patients with fever and meningitis symptoms require antibiotics immediately. Do not wait for the LP kit. Give the antibiotics, then approach the LP.

- Consider changing or removing Foley catheters and any indwelling IV sites.

SHORTNESS OF BREATH

... You were in good physical shape ...

What are the patient's vital signs, including temperature? When was the onset of SOB and what was the reason for admission? Does the patient have COPD or is the patient getting oxygen?

Order oxygen and an ABG kit to the bedside. Patients with SOB need to be seen immediately.

Major Causes of Shortness of Breath

Pulmonary: Asthma, COPD, pulmonary embolism, pneumonia
Cardiovascular: CHF, cardiac tamponade
Others: Pneumothorax, obstruction (e.g. mucus plug), anxiety

Things You Don't Want to Miss (Call Your Resident)

Inadequate tissue oxygenation (i.e., hypoxia)

Key History

- Check BP, pulse, respirations, O_2 saturations, and temperature.
- Quickly look at the patient and review the chart. Get an ECG, ABG, and CXR if the patient looks sick.

Focused Examination

	KEY POINTS
General	How distressed or sick does the patient look?
Vitals	Repeat now. Check for a pulsus paradoxus.
Neurologic	Mentation and check for central cyanosis.
Cardiovascular	Heart rate, jugular venous pulse, skin temperature and color, capillary refill.
Lungs	Listen for crackles and breath sounds on both sides, evidence of consolidation or effusion.

Laboratory Data

Consider ABG, ECG, troponins, CBC, D-dimer, V/Q scan, and CXR.

Management

- Order empiric oxygen to keep saturations >92%. Be cautious if the patient has COPD and is a retainer of CO_2—in that case, keep O_2 saturations around 88% to 90% and check ABG. Remember that the O_2 saturation tells you nothing about pH or Pco_2.

- For asthma or COPD, administer albuterol and ipatropium by nebulizer, q2–4h until stable. Consider IV corticosteroids, methylprednisolone (Solu-Medrol), 60 mg IV q6h, and antibiotics if needed.

- For CHF, is the patient volume overloaded? Raise the head of the patient's bed. Administer furosemide (Lasix), 20–40 mg IV, and albuterol nebulizer. Consider morphine or nitroglycerin. Assess for adequate diuresis.

- For suspected cardiac tamponade, order a stat cardiac echo and cardiology consult.

- For pulmonary embolism, often the patient is tachycardic and tachypneic and has a sudden onset of SOB. The classic ECG is S_1, Q_3, and T_3 (S waves in lead I, Q waves in lead III, inverted T waves in lead III). If suspicion is high, consider starting heparin or LMWH. Ensure that the patient has no history of bleeding disorders, PUD, recent CVA, or surgery. Obtain a V/Q scan or spiral CT. Also, consider lower extremity Dopplers and D-dimer.

- Acute respiratory failure is generally defined by ABG of P_{O_2} <60 or P_{CO_2} >50 with a pH <7.30 while on room air. Ensure that the patient hasn't received narcotics recently. If so, consider naloxone, 0.2 mg IV. Acute respiratory acidosis with a pH <7.20 usually requires mechanical ventilation.

GASTROINTESTINAL BLEEDING

... Ahh, the smell of melena ...

What are the patient's vital signs? When was the onset of bleeding and what is the reason for admission? Is the bleeding upper (coffee ground emesis, melena) or lower (hematochezia)? How much blood has been lost?

 Confirm that the patient has IV access (at least 18 gauge) and recent CBC. Type and cross-match blood. If the patient is tachycardic or hypotensive, see the patient immediately.

Major Causes of Gastrointestinal Bleeding

- Upper: Esophageal varices, Mallory-Weiss tear, peptic ulcer, esophagitis, neoplasm, aortoenteric fistula (history of AAA repair)

- Lower: Diverticulosis, angiodysplasia, neoplasm, IBD, infectious colitis, anorectal disease (hemorrhoids, fissures)

Things You Don't Want to Miss (Call Your Resident)

GI bleeding leading to hypovolemic shock.

Key History

- Check BP, pulse, respirations, O_2 saturations, and temperature. Orthostatic BP.

- Quickly look at the patient and review the chart.

Focused Examination

	KEY POINTS
General	How distressed or sick does the patient look?
Vitals	Repeat now.
Neurologic	Mentation.
Cardiovascular	Heart rate, jugular venous pulse, skin temperature and color, capillary refill.
Abdomen	Check for tenderness, bowel sounds, look for ascites.
Rectal	Must be performed; guaiac stool.

Laboratory Data

Consider CBC, coags, and CMP.

Management

- Insert two large-bore IVs (16–18 gauge), type and cross pRBCs. It can take up to 8 hours for CBC to equilibrate, so initial Hct may be falsely elevated. In absence of renal disease, high BUN suggests GI bleeding. Check coags and platelets to exclude bleeding disorders. Is the patient receiving anticoagulants? If so, stop the anticoagulant and consider reversal with vitamin K or FFP.

- Consider whether special blood products are required based on comorbidities (e.g., irradiated, washed RBCs). Also consider whether the patient needs premedication with acetaminophen/diphenhydramine based on prior transfusions.

- Replenish the intravascular volume by giving IV fluids (normal saline), especially while awaiting blood products. Keep the patient NPO.

- For upper GI bleeding, insert a nasogastric tube to assess if active bleeding is present. Suppress acid with omeprazole, 40 mg PO bid. GI consult for endoscopy. If bleeding has stopped and the patient is hemodynamically stable, elective endoscopy can be performed within the next 24 hours. Otherwise, urgent endoscopy may be required.

- For active variceal bleeding, start octreotide, 50 μg bolus, then 50 μg/hour, correct coagulation deficits, replace pRBCs as needed. Call a GI consult as urgent endoscopy may be required.

- For lower GI bleeding, correct fluid status. If hemodynamically stable, obtain GI consult for colonoscopy. If unstable, an urgent tagged RBC scan should be scheduled. Also, consider arteriography.

- Surgery consult/indications include the following:

  1. Aortoenteric fistula.

  2. Uncontrollable or recurrent bleeding.

  3. Bleeding episode requiring transfusion of more than 6 units pRBCs.

  4. Visible naked vessel seen in peptic ulcer by endoscopy.

13

Common Calls and Complaints

... Call me again. Go ahead, make my day ...

ALCOHOL WITHDRAWAL

Alcohol withdrawal can be a problem both medically and behaviorally. The biggest danger is delirium tremens (DTs), which has up to a 15% mortality rate and requires close monitoring. Watch for DT symptoms of confusion, tachycardia, dilated pupils, and diaphoresis, usually 2 to 7 days after the last drink, although other symptoms can occur before then. DTs should be managed with sedatives promptly. IV fluids and electrolyte repletion are also helpful. If the patient is not in imminent danger but is symptomatic, consider management with the following steps until substance abuse treatment can be arranged:

- Place the patient in an environment where the patient is not endangering him- or herself or others.

- Consider lorazepam (Ativan), 0.5–1 mg PO/IV/IM q6–8h (scheduled or prn) or chlordiazepoxide (Librium), 100 mg PO tid, for symptoms of withdrawal. Use sitter or restraints as necessary.

- Thiamine, 100 mg PO/IV/IM q day, and folate, 1 mg PO q day, can be given as preventive measures.

   Strongly encourage the patient to seek substance abuse treatment and counseling. Social workers can assist with suggestions, and chemical dependency consultation can also be arranged for inpatient and outpatient detoxification. See also Chemical Dependency section in Chapter 17.

BLEEDING AT LINE SITES AND AFTER PROCEDURES

Bleeding at central line sites is a common problem. Consider oozing, coagulation disorders, antiplatelet and anticoagulation drugs as causes of bleeding. Confirm that bleeding does not extend into the soft tissues of the neck, causing upper airway obstruction. If so, an emergent ENT consult should be called. Otherwise, consider the following steps:

- Under sterile conditions, remove the dressing and apply continuous pressure (no peeking!) to the entry site for 15 minutes. If the bleeding has stopped, clean the site and apply occlusive dressing. If bleeding has not stopped, suspect a coagulation disorder. A single suture may help provide hemostasis.

- When bleeding occurs after cardiac catheterization, the cardiology fellow should be notified immediately. Initial management can be occlusive pressure and sandbag. Consider obtaining a CBC and a noncontrast abdominal CT to evaluate for a retroperitoneal hematoma if there is protracted bleeding and/or hemodynamic compromise.

CONSTIPATION

Constipation is one of the most common complaints or calls of hospitalized patients and is something you can usually handle over the telephone. Make sure the patient isn't having N/V, abdominal pain, or fecal impaction. If these are suspected, you must see the patient. Otherwise, consider the following agents:

- Docusate (Colace), 100 mg PO bid (stool softener). Consider giving as prevention to any patient on narcotics or bedridden patients. Usually doesn't produce the necessary effect desired unless used prophylactically.

- Senna (Senokot), 2 tablets PO up to four times a day prn or senna/docusate (Senna-S), 2 tablets PO bid prn.

- Bisacodyl (Dulcolax), 10 mg PO/PR prn (stimulant).

- Consider enemas if oral agents have not been effective. Fleets or tap water enemas can be used. Do not order enemas in a neutropenic patient.

If the above don't work, consider:

- Lactulose, 30 cc PO q4–6h until bowel movement.

- Polyethylene glycol (Miralax), 17 g dissolved in 4–8 oz H_2O PO q day.

- Magnesium citrate 150–300 mL PO q day-bid.

COUGH

Cough is one of the most irritating symptoms both for the patient and the house officer. Make sure the patient isn't having massive hemoptysis (defined as >600 mL over 48 hours or enough to impair gas exchange) and try to diagnose the underlying cause. Symptomatically, consider the following steps:

- Guaifenesin/dextromethorphan or codeine (Robitussin DM or AC), 10 mL PO q4h prn

- Codeine, 10–20 mg PO q4–6h prn.

- Benzonatate capsules (Tessalon Perles), 100 mg PO tid.

DIARRHEA

Diarrhea is defined as increasing frequency and/or increasing fluidity of stools. Acute diarrhea is frequently self-limited. Determine extent of associated symptoms (N/V, blood in stools, abdominal pain). Don't forget the possibility of ischemic colitis and fecal impaction with overflow incontinence. Be careful about patients on corticosteroids with minimal abdominal symptoms having an intra-abdominal process.

Consider the following items:

- NPO with IV hydration.

- Consider correcting electrolytes.

- Discontinue possible causes including laxatives, antibiotics, antacids with magnesium.

- Consider checking CBC, stool samples (for WBC, culture and sensitivity, ova and parasites), and *C. difficile* toxin (especially if there has been recent antibiotic use) if indicated.

- Loperamide, 4 mg initially, and then 2 mg PO with each loose bowel movement. Be cautious with infectious colitis.

- Bismuth subsalicylate (Pepto-Bismol), 30 mL PO q6h.

FALLS

This is a call where you must go see the patient. Find out from the patient what occurred and where the patient is having pain. Also talk with witnesses. Ask nursing for a bedside glucose test and vital signs. Examine the patient, including a careful neurological exam, and look for any signs of injury. Clearly document what occurred in the patient's chart. Other steps to consider:

- If you have any concerns about head trauma or note a change in mental status or the patient is on anticoagulants or has a coagulopathy, check a stat head CT without contrast to rule out a bleed.

- Check recent lab results and ECG/telemetry. Consider checking films for possible trauma.

- Look at the medication list for possible contributing factors (sedatives, antihypertensives, hypoglycemic agents).

- Place patient on fall precautions. Consider q2 hour neurological checks by nursing for the next 12–24 hours in patients with head injuries.

HYPERGLYCEMIA AND HYPOGLYCEMIA

Hyperglycemia

The severity should be determined by the glucose level and patient's symptoms. Confirm that the patient is not receiving IV fluids containing glucose. Most type 2 diabetics should be on a scheduled sliding scale insulin dose. A conservative scale is as follows, with Accuchecks qid:

Glucose	Regular insulin subcut
60–200	0 units
201–250	2 units
251–300	4 units
301–350	6 units
351–400	8 units
>400	10 units and call house officer
<60	1 Amp D50 IV and call house officer. If taking PO, can give PO juice/crackers, etc.

- Severe hyperglycemia with DKA is a medical emergency and is not covered here.
- All type 1 diabetics require scheduled dosages of insulin, even if they are NPO. Give $\frac{1}{2}$ to $\frac{2}{3}$ of usual basal insulin dose to patients who are NPO. If patient will be NPO >24 hours, consider starting IV insulin and IV glucose drips and titrate to keep blood glucose between 100–200.

Hypoglycemia

Any symptomatic patient with hypoglycemia should be treated.

- For mild hypoglycemia in an awake patient, oral sweetened juices can be given.
- With increasing severity, or if the patient is not able to take PO, D50 should be given IV (1 Amp).
- If IV access is unavailable with severe hypoglycemia, glucagon, 1 mg subcut, or IM can be given.
- Review the patient's medications for medications causing hypoglycemia (oral hypoglycemics, quinine, sulfa drugs).
- If ongoing hypoglycemia occurs or the patient is NPO, start a maintenance D5W infusion at 75–100 mL/hr.

HOLDING MEDICATIONS FOR MORNING TESTS

Many tests require that patients are NPO. Always consider making patient's NPO after midnight if there is potential for testing the following day. Most orders are written NPO after midnight except medications. Certain tests (cardiac stress tests) require that you also hold β-blockers and calcium channel blockers the morning of the test. Hold metformin (Glucophage) 24 hours prior to studies involving IV iodinated contrast. If the test is canceled, make sure to restart the diet. For specific recommendations, please refer to Preparation for Radiologic and Endoscopic Procedures (see Chap. 16).

INSOMNIA

Insomnia is a common problem in the hospital. The patient's mental status must be considered before administering medications. Make sure delirium and dementia aren't present as well as pain that may be keeping the patient awake.

Otherwise, consider use of the following agents:

- Antihistamines such as diphenhydramine (Benadryl), 25 mg PO qhs prn. Be conscious of anticholinergic side effects, especially in the elderly.

- Zolpidem (Ambien) or zaleplon (Sonata), 5–10 mg PO qhs prn.

- Benzodiazepines, such as temazepam (Restoril), 15–30 mg PO qhs prn.

LACK OF INTRAVENOUS ACCESS

Determine if IV access is necessary (i.e., essential IV medications such as antibiotics, transfusions, etc.). Consider if IV medications can be given orally.

If access is necessary, see the patient and attempt peripheral line placement. If not successful, call IV therapy for assistance. Then consider other types of access such as PICC lines. If these are not options, consider central venous access. Please refer to Guide to Procedures (see Chap. 18).

NAUSEA AND VOMITING

Nausea and vomiting are always a symptom of an underlying etiology (like having eaten hospital food on- or postcall). While working up the underlying cause and eliminating life-threatening etiologies, consider using the following agents:

- Prochlorperazine (Compazine), 5–10 mg IV/PO/IM q4–6h prn (also in suppository form, 25 mg bid).

- Promethazine (Phenergan), 25 mg PO/IM/PR q4–6h prn.

- Metoclopramide (Reglan), 10 mg PO/IV/IM q6h prn.

- Trimethobenzamide (Tigan), 250 mg PO q6–8h prn.

- Odansetron (Zofran), 4–8 mg PO/IV q8h prn.

PRURITUS

While identifying the underlying cause, consider the use of the following agents:

- Diphenhydramine (Benadryl), 25–50 mg PO q6–8h prn or nonsedating antihistamine such as fexofenadine (Allegra), 180 mg PO q day.

- Hydroxyzine (Atarax, Vistaril), 25 mg PO q6–8h prn.

- Sarna lotion.

- For refractory pruritis, consider doxepin 5% cream q 3–4 hours prn or doxepin 25 mg PO q day (short-term use only).

RASH

First, make sure that this is not an *anaphylactic* reaction. Specifically look for an urticarial rash with associated SOB, wheezing, laryngeal edema, and hypotension. If these symptoms are present, consider the following items:

- Large-bore (16 gauge) access for IV fluids.

- Epinephrine, 0.5 mg (1:1,000 solution) IV or subcut.

- Diphenhydramine (Benadryl), 50 mg IV or 50–100 mg IM.

- Hydrocortisone, 500 mg IV or methylprednisolone 125 mg IV.

- Albuterol 2.5 mg by nebulizer can be administered for bronchospasm.

- Intubation if the airway is compromised.

The most common cause of rashes in-house is a *drug reaction*. Hold medication that may be the cause if this is not an essential medication. Consider a dermatology or allergy consult (for desensitization) in the AM if the medication is necessary. For symptomatic relief:

- Diphenhydramine (Benadryl), 25–50 mg PO q6–8h prn; hydroxyzine (Atarax), 25 mg PO q6–8h prn; fexofenadine (Allegra), 180 mg PO q day; or loratadine (Claritin), 10 mg PO q day if itching is present.

- Corticosteroid creams.

- Consider PO steroids such as prednisone, if severe.

SUNDOWNING

This is a common call overnight. Risk factors for sundowning include increased age, dementia, and ICU admission. The patient can present with confusion, disorientation, or combativeness in the evening hours. Things to consider:

- Identify and treat any underlying conditions that could be contributing.

- Minimize sedation. If absolutely necessary, haloperidol (Haldol), 0.25 mg PO/IM q day or risperidone (Risperdal) 0.5 mg PO qpm; increase as needed.

- Maintain a quiet structured environment to help calm the patient down. Provide frequent reorientation; family members can be helpful in this respect.

- Consider a sitter or a bed alarm if the patient wanders. Avoid restraints if possible as they can worsen agitation and confusion.

TRANSFUSION REACTIONS

If an **acute hemolytic reaction** is suspected, follow these steps:

- Immediately stop the transfusion and send bags and patient's blood sample to the laboratory for testing, including cross-match, Coombs' test, CBC, DIC panel, total bilirubin, and BMP.

- Rehydrate with intravascular fluid.

- Closely monitor renal function, electrolytes (especially K), and coags.

- Keep urine output >100 mL/hr.

If **severe, nonhemolytic reaction** is suspected (including anaphylactic symptoms, wheezing, respiratory distress, temperature >40°C):

- D/C transfusion and send bag and line for repeat cross-match.

- Consider diphenhydramine, 25–50 mg PO/IV.

- Consider hydrocortisone, 500 mg IV.

- Consider epinephrine, 0.5–1.0 mL (1:1,000) IM.

For **volume overload**:

- Decrease rate of transfusion.

- Consider furosemide, 20–40 mg IV.

For **fever <40°C or chills**:

- Slow down rate of transfusion.

- Acetaminophen, 650 mg PO.

- Meperidine 20–50 mg IV can be used for chills.

- Continue monitoring.

14   Pain Control

... As if anything could control your pain ...

GENERAL POINTS

- Treating undiagnosed pain can be perilous: always have a plan under way to diagnose the source and type of pain you are treating.

- Pain is often an undertreated symptom; once a diagnosis is made, the patient should have enough pain medications to keep him or her comfortable.

- Scheduled pain medications at appropriate doses are a viable alternative to try before switching or adding medications.

- Standing pain medication orders (can write: "patient can refuse" or "for breakthrough pain") can minimize phone calls and interrupted sleep. You will want to be notified if the patient's pain or symptoms(s) persist or worsen as this may signal a change in the patient's condition.

- Consider getting an anesthesia or pain consult for other options in persistent, severe, uncontrolled pain.

- Before prescribing pain medications, always consider comorbidities, allergies, drug interactions, and potential side effects.

- Trust your instincts. If you think a patient is manipulative and drug-seeking, set your boundaries and stick with them. Questions to ask:

    1. Does the patient only ask for pain medications when you are in the room?

    2. Do others observe different behaviors when you leave the room?

    3. Is the patient talking or resting comfortably?

    4. Is the patient allergic to every pain medication except the one he or she is requesting?

TABLE 14-1.
SELECTED AGENTS IN THE THREE-STEP ANALGESIC LADDER

Agent	Oral	Parenteral
Step 1. Mild pain: nonopioid		
Acetaminophen	650 mg q4–6h PRN or 1,000 mg q6h PRN	—
Aspirin	650 mg q4–6h PRN or 1,000 mg q6h PRN	—
Ibuprofen	400–800 mg q6–8h PRN	—
Gabapentin (for neuropathic pain)	Start 300 mg qhs	—
Step 2. Moderate pain: weak opioid (± nonopioid)		
Tylenol #3 (codeine 30 mg/ acetaminophen 300 mg)	1–2 tablets PO q4h PRN	—
Percocet (oxycodone 5 mg/ acetaminophen 325 mg)	1–2 tablets q4–6h PRN	—
Oxycodone	5 mg q4–6h	—
Tramadol	50–100 mg q4–6h (maximum, 400 mg/day)	—
Step 3. Severe pain: strong opioid (± nonopioid)		
Morphine	10–30 mg q3–4h (around the clock or in-termittent dosing)	0.1–0.2 mg/kg (up to 15 mg) q4h
Morphine (controlled release)	Can start 30 mg q8–12h and increase PRN to 90–120 mg q12h	—
Fentanyl[a]	—	0.1 mg q1–3h
Hydromorphone	2–4 mg q4–6h	1–4 mg q4–6h
Levorphanol	2 mg q6–8h	2 mg q6–8h
Oxymorphone	—	1 mg q3–4h

(Continued)

TABLE 14-1.
SELECTED AGENTS IN THE THREE-STEP ANALGESIC
LADDER (Continued)

Agent	Oral	Parenteral
Morphine PCA pump	—	1 mg/hr basal rate, 1 mg q15 minute lockout, but individualize per patient

[a] Transdermal fentanyl: 100 μg/hr = 315–404 mg/day of oral morphine and 53–67 mg/day of IM morphine.

All medications in PO form unless otherwise denoted.

Consider giving a stool softener daily with sustained narcotic use.

Adapted from Jacox et al, 1994, and World Health Organization, 1996.

15

Therapeutic Considerations

... Dose, trough, peak—just a therapeutic level I seek ...

Antibiotics and anticoagulation are two of the most common therapeutics in the hospital setting.

ANTIBIOTICS
General Points

Three main issues must be addressed when selecting antibiotics:

1. Expected pathogen and patient demographics (i.e., nosocomial, immunocompromised).

2. Patient allergies.

3. Renal and hepatic function.

See *The Sanford Guide to Antimicrobial Therapy* for specific choices by site as well as renal dose adjustments and drug interactions.

Some Specifics on Commonly Used Antibiotics
Vancomycin

Use in severe gram-positive infections or MRSA/ORSA. The dose is based on body weight, whereas the dosing interval is based on creatinine clearance.

BODY WEIGHT (KG)	DOSE (MG)
<45	500
45–60	750
61–90	1,000
>90	1,250–1,500

CRCL (ML/MIN)	INTERVAL
>60	12 hrs
35–60	24 hrs
15–34	48 hrs
<15	Random dosing

- Drug levels are not recommended for patients receiving a short course of therapy (<5 days).

- Periodic trough levels (every week) are recommended in patients receiving longer courses of therapy to ensure concentrations are adequate. Trough levels should be obtained approximately 30 minutes before the next dose. Therapeutic trough levels range from 5–15 mg/L. Peak levels are generally not of benefit. Hemodialysis patients should have a serum drug level measured every 4–7 days to determine timing of subsequent doses.

- Serum creatinine should be monitored weekly.

Aminoglycosides

Aminoglycosides are active against aerobic gram-negative bacteria. Synergistic with β-lactam antibiotics. Adverse effects include ototoxicity, nephrotoxicity, and neuromuscular paralysis.

Extended interval (i.e., infrequent dosing) regimens are generally recommended. Exceptions include pregnancy, dialysis, CrCl <20, and endocarditis, where traditional-based dosing is recommended.

Extended Interval Aminoglycoside Nomogram (Figure 15-1)

- Initial dose:

    Gentamicin, 5 mg/kg
    Tobramycin, 5 mg/kg
    Amikacin, 15 mg/kg

- Use IBW to calculate dose.

    For men: IBW = 50 kg + 2.3 (height [inches] − 60)

    For women: IBW = 45.5 kg + 2.3 (height [inches] − 60)

    If >20% above IBW, use formula IBW + 0.4 (actual body weight − IBW)

CRCL (mL/MIN)	INTERVAL
>60	24 hrs
40–59	36 hrs
20–39	48 hrs
<20	Use traditional dosing

- Obtain midinterval drug level 8–12 hours after the initial dose, then evaluate based on nomogram.

- Repeat drug level 1–2 times weekly and monitor serum creatinine 2–3 times weekly.

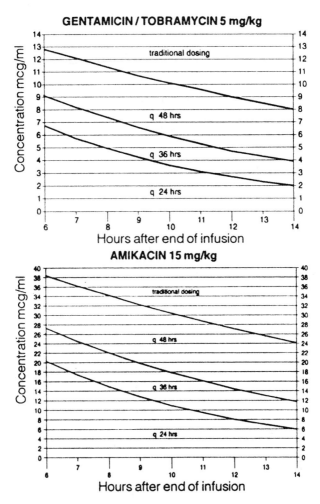

FIGURE 15-1. Extended interval aminoglycoside nomogram. (From Barnes-Jewish Hospital Department of Pharmacy. St. Louis: Washington University Medical Center, 1996.)

Traditional Aminoglycoside Dosing
• Loading Dose

- Gentamicin, tobramycin

  For urinary tract infection or synergy against gram-positive cocci (GPC): 1–1.5 mg/kg
  For systemic illness: 2 mg/kg
  For critical illness/sepsis 2.5 mg/kg

- Amikacin

  5–7.5 mg/kg dose based on levels

Maintenance doses: See Figure 15-2. Check aminoglycoside trough immediately before third dose and aminoglycoside peak 1 hour after start of third infusion. Peaks should be 3–5 μg/mL (UTI, synergy against GPC) or 6–10 μg/mL (systemic or critical illness). Troughs should be <2 μg/mL.

Maintenance dose is a PERCENTAGE of the selected loading dose. Example: 70 kg pt with CrCl=60mL/min and pneumonia. LD=140mg, MD=120mg q12h.

CrCl (mL/min)	t1/2 (hr)	q8h	q12h	q24h
>90	3.1	84%	100%	-
80	3.4	80%	91%	-
70	3.9	76%	88%	-
60	4.5	-	84%	-
50	5.3	-	79%	-
40	6.5	-	-	92%
30	8.4	-	-	86%
25	9.9	-	-	81%
20	11.9	-	-	75%

For CrCl < 20 ml/min, give loading dose, then follow levels and redose when level drops below 2mcg/ml.

FIGURE 15-2. Traditional nomogram. (From Barnes-Jewish Hospital Department of Pharmacy. St. Louis: Washington University Medical Center, 1996.)

ANTICOAGULATION

... No bleed should be your creed ...

Before initiating anticoagulant therapy, ensure that the patient has no history of active peptic ulcers, recent stroke or bleeding, or recent surgery. All patients should have a digital rectal examination and documented guaiac status.

Heparin Weight-Based Dosing (Unfractionated)

• Initial bolus—round to the nearest 100 units.

Acute MI: 60 units/kg, maximum 4,000 units.
DVT/PE: 80 units/kg, no maximum.
Non-DVT/PE or acute MI: 60 units/kg, maximum of 5,000 units.
High risk of bleeding: Consider smaller bolus.

• IV Infusion rate.

Acute MI: 12 units/kg/hr, maximum 1,000 units/hr.
DVT/PE: 18 units/kg/hr.
Non-DVT/PE or acute MI: 14 units/kg/hr.
High risk of bleeding: 12 units/kg/hr.

An activated PTT should be ordered 6 hours after initial bolus and 6 hours after each rate change. After two consecutive aPTTs are therapeutic (60–94 secs), the aPTT should be monitored each morning. In addition, CBC with platelets should be monitored every 48 hours while on IV heparin.

Heparin nomogram

aPTT (sec)*	Bolus	Infusion rate
<40	3,000 units	Increase by 3 units/kg/hr
40–50	2,000 units	Increase by 2 units/kg/hr
51–59	None	Increase by 1 unit/kg/hr
60–94	None	No change
95–104	None	Decrease by 1 unit/kg/hr
105–114	Hold for 30 minutes	Decrease by 2 units/kg/hr
>114	Hold for 1 hr	Decrease by 3 units/kg/hr

*Note: Activated partial thromboplastin time (aPTT) can vary depending on lab; check local scale.

Low Molecular Weight Heparin Dosing

- **Enoxaparin** 1 mg/kg subcutaneously q12h (unstable angina or DVT).

- **Dalteparin** 120 units/kg subcutaneously q12h (unstable angina) or 200 units/kg subcutaneously q12h (DVT).

- **Tinzaparin** 175 anti Xa units/kg subcutaneously q day (DVT).

- Dosages need to be adjusted in patients with renal failure; unfractionated heparin is recommended for patients with a CrCl <10 or on hemodialysis. Antifactor Xa can be checked in patients with CrCl <30 mL/min. Risk of bleeding is increased in patients with antifactor Xa levels above 0.8 units/mL.

Warfarin nomogram (for starting warfarin therapy)

DAY	INR	DOSAGE (MG)
1	—	5
2	<1.5	5
	1.5–1.9	2.5
	2–2.5	1–2.5
	>2.5	0
3	<1.5	5–10
	1.5–1.9	2.5–5
	2–3	0–2.5
	>3	0
4	<1.5	10
	1.5–1.9	5–7.5
	2–3	0–5
	>3	0
5	<1.5	10
	1.5–1.9	7.5–10
	2–3	0–5
	>3	0

From Andritsos L, Yusen RD, Eby C. Disorders of Hemostasis. In *Washington Manual of Medical Therapeutics, 31st edition.* Lippincott, Williams & Wilkins, 2004.

Note: Warfarin affects the CYP450 system and therefore has numerous drug interactions; consider monitoring levels of drugs metabolized by the CYP450 system while patient is on warfarin.

Guidelines for Antithrombotic Therapy

- **Atrial fibrillation/atrial flutter**, goal INR 2-3.

  1. For cardioversion, if rhythm has been present >48 hours, anticoagulate for 3 weeks prior to procedure and 4 weeks afterwards.

  2. For rate-controlled patients—lifelong.

  3. For patients at low risk (no h/o CVA, TIA, HTN, DM, heart disease, age <75 years) or in patients in whom warfarin therapy is contraindicated, consider ASA 325 mg q day only.

- **DVT/PE**, goal INR 2–3.

  1. First episode—6–12 months.

  2. >1 episode—lifelong.

- **Tissue or St. Judes valve in aortic position**, goal INR 2–3.

  1. Tissue—3 months.

  2. St. Judes in aortic position—lifelong.

- **Mechanical valve** (except St. Judes in aortic position), goal INR 2.5–3.5.

  1. Mechanical—lifelong.

  2. Consider adding ASA for caged-ball or caged disc valves, if h/o CAD, embolism, or mitral valve replacement.

Treatment of High INR
INR <5 Without Bleeding

- Hold warfarin for 1 dose or lower dose, search for occult bleed, D/C all other antithrombotic/antiplatelet therapy, and follow INR until back in therapeutic range.

INR 5–9 Without Bleeding

- Hold warfarin for 1–2 doses and monitor INR; can also administer vitamin K_1, 1–2.5 mg PO if at increased risk of bleeding or patient requires urgent surgery. Document decrease in INR within 48 hours. Give additional vitamin K_1 if INR remains high.

INR >9 Without Bleeding

- Hold warfarin; give vitamin K_1, 5–10 mg PO; follow INR every 8 hours, and repeat vitamin K_1 as needed.

- Consider admitting the patient if close follow-up is not possible.

Minor Bleeding

- Hold warfarin; give vitamin K_1, 1–5 mg PO; follow INR every 8 hours, and repeat vitamin K as needed. If bleeding not controlled, treat as for major bleeding.

Major Bleeding

- Hold warfarin; admit patient; give vitamin K_1, 10 mg IV, and FFP; follow INR every 6 hours; and repeat vitamin K_1 q12h until INR <1.3 or bleeding has stopped. Control bleeding as needed through transfusions, surgery, etc.

Notes:

- Vitamin K_1 can be given in equivalent dosages PO, subcutaneously, or IVPB. Oral administration is preferred for nonlife-threatening bleeding; IV administration should be reserved for major bleeding. The response to subcutaneous administration is less predictable, but it is still effective.

- If vitamin K_1 is given IVPB, administer slowly to minimize risk of anaphylactoid reaction.

16

Tools of the Trade (Fluids, Electrolytes, Vital Signs, Electrocardiography, Radiology)

FLUIDS AND BASIC ELECTROLYTES
Basal Requirements

... To start 'em up ...

Water

- Basal water requirement may be calculated as follows:

  For the first 10 kg of body weight, 4 mL/kg/hr plus,
  for the second 10 kg of body weight, 2 mL/kg/hr plus,
  for remaining weight above 20 kg, 1 mL/kg/hr.

- Fever, increased respiratory rate, and sweating can all increase insensible water losses. Insensible losses increase by 100–150 mL/day for each degree of body temperature above 37°C.

Electrolytes

- Sodium: 50–150 mmol/day (as NaCl). Most of this is excreted in the urine.

- Chloride: 50–150 mmol/day (as NaCl).

- Potassium: 20–60 mmol/day (as KCl), assuming renal function is normal. Most of this is excreted in the urine.

Carbohydrates

- Dextrose, 100–150 g/day.

- IV dextrose administration minimizes protein catabolism and prevents ketoacidosis.

Maintenance Intravenous Fluids

... To keep 'em going ...

- Basal requirements of water, electrolytes, and carbohydrates can be conveniently administered as 0.45% NaCl in 5% dextrose plus 20 mmol/L KCl.

- Fluid losses can be divided as urinary losses and all other losses. Urinary losses for the average adult are 0.5–1 mL/kg/hr (e.g., 70 kg person produces approximately 40–60 mL/hr or 1,200 mL/day). Other losses (water lost in sweat, stool, hydration, insensible losses) total approximately 800 cc/day.

- For average sized adults, 2–3 L (90–125 mL/hr) of this IV solution per day is sufficient (i.e., $D_5\frac{1}{2}$ NS + 20 mEq KCl @ 100 mL/hr).

- Patients with hypovolemia require more aggressive fluid resuscitation, generally with 0.9% NaCl. Patients with renal failure or CHF may require less.

- GI and renal losses may significantly increase the loss of water, Na^+, and K^+. Serum electrolytes should be followed closely in these situations.

ELECTROLYTE ABNORMALITIES

… If it's high, lower it. If it's low, get it back up …

Hyponatremia

… Please pass the salt …

Etiology

- **Hypotonic hyponatremia** is usually caused by primary water gain or Na^+ loss. Na^+ loss may be the result of renal or extrarenal causes.

- **Hypertonic hyponatremia** is caused by an increase in extracellular solute concentration (e.g., hyperglycemia or IV mannitol administration).

- **Isotonic hyponatremia** (**pseudohyponatremia**) occurs as a result of a decrease in the aqueous phase of plasma (e.g., hyperproteinemia, hyperlipidemia). The concentration of Na^+ per liter of plasma water is normal.

Evaluation

- A careful H&P should be done, paying close attention to fluid status and the neurologic examination.

- Plasma osmolality, urine osmolality, and urine Na^+ should be measured.

- Refer to Figure 16-1.

Treatment

- Mild asymptomatic hyponatremia generally requires no treatment.

- For isovolemic and hypervolemic hypotonic hyponatremia, consider fluid restriction.

- For hypovolemic hypotonic hyponatremia, consider saline therapy.

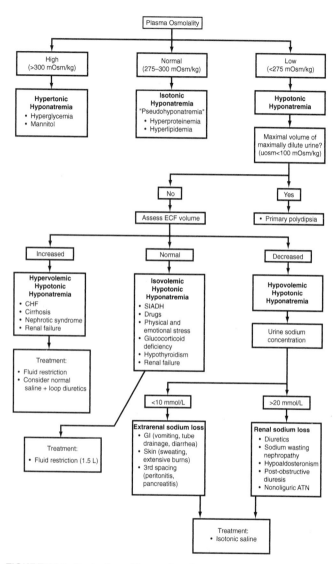

FIGURE 16-1. Evaluation of hyponatremia.

- Careful consideration should be given to the rate of correction of the serum $[Na^+]$. Too rapid correction may result in osmotic demyelination or central pontine myelinolysis.

- Rapidly developing hyponatremia tends to develop with CNS symptoms and requires more rapid correction. **Severe** symptomatic hyponatremia should be treated with hypertonic saline. The rate of increase of the plasma $[Na^+]$ should not exceed 1–2 mmol/L/hr and no more than 8 mmol/L in the first 24 hours.

- If acute or severe with symptoms, correct $[Na^+]$ to 120–125 in first 24 hours, usually with hypertonic saline, and then gradually until completely corrected over 3–5 days.

- The quantity of $[Na^+]$ required to increase the plasma $[Na^+]$ by a given amount can be estimated as follows:

$$[Na^+] \text{ deficit (mmol)} = \text{desired change in } [Na^+] \times TBW$$

$$TBW = 0.6 \times \text{body weight (kg)}.$$

- For example, if the desired change in $[Na^+]$ is 8 mmol in a 70 kg patient, then 336 mmol of $[Na^+]$ would be required ($42 \times 8 = 336$). This would be 0.65 L hypertonic (3%) saline (336 mmol ÷ 513 mmol/L) or 2.2 L isotonic (0.9%) saline (336 mmol ÷ 154 mmol/L).

Hypernatremia

... Hold the salt ...

Etiology

- Hypernatremia is caused by Na^+ gain or water deficit.

- **Water deficit caused by decreased intake** may be seen in patients with limited access to water (e.g., mental status alteration, intubated patients) or impaired thirst.

- **Water loss may be the result of renal or extrarenal causes.**

- Rarely, hypernatremia may result from **excess Na$^+$ intake** (e.g., hypertonic saline or $NaHCO_3$).

Evaluation

- A careful H&P should be done, paying close attention to fluid status and the neurologic examination.

- Plasma osmolality, urine osmolality, and urine $[Na^+]$ should be measured.

- Solute excretion rate = urine osmolality × urine volume.

- Refer to Figure 16-2.

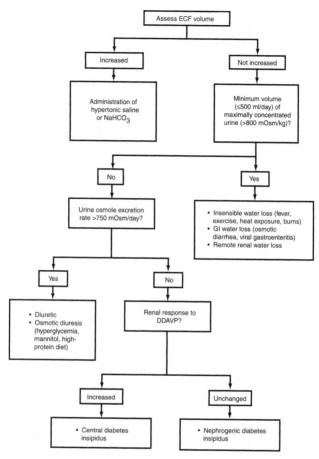

FIGURE 16-2. Evaluation of hypernatremia.

Treatment

- Underlying conditions should be treated (e.g., hyperglycemia, diarrhea, etc.).

- ECF volume should be restored in hypovolemic patients with isotonic saline.

$$\text{Body water deficit (L)} = \frac{(\text{plasma } [Na^+] - 140)}{140} \times \text{TBW (L)}$$

$$\text{TBW} = 0.6 \times \text{body weight (kg)}$$

- As with hyponatremia, too rapid correction of hypernatremia is potentially dangerous. The rate of correction of the plasma $[Na^+]$ should not exceed 0.5 mmol/L/hr and the $[Na^+]$ should decrease by no more than 12 mmol/L over the first 24 hours (or no faster than one-half of the volume deficit in the initial 24 hours).

- Don't forget to take into account ongoing losses. The safest route is PO or NG tube administration of water. Alternatively, one-half NS (0.45%), one-quarter NS (0.225%), or D5W can be given IV. Reassess volume status and Na every 8–12 hours.

- Central diabetes insipidus is treated with intranasal DDAVP.

- Nephrogenic diabetes insipidus may be reversible by treating the underlying disorder or eliminating the offending drug (e.g., lithium).

Hypokalemia

... More bananas, please ...

- Defined as a $[K^+]$ <3.5 mmol/L, the clinical features vary greatly. Myalgias and weakness are common complaints. Severe hypokalemia can result in an increased risk of arrhythmias. The $[K^+]$ level of cardiac patients is generally maintained above 4.

Etiology

- Hypokalemia may be caused by **decreased intake**. It is infrequently the sole cause but can exacerbate other causes of hypokalemia.

- **Intracellular shifts** (metabolic alkalosis, insulin, stress-induced catecholamine release, β-adrenergic agonists, anabolic states) may result in hypokalemia.

- K^+ depletion may also be caused by **nonrenal and renal loss**. Renal loss of K^+ may be caused by increased distal K^+ secretion or increased distal tubular flow rate. Diuretics (thiazides and loop) are a common cause. GI causes include vomiting and diarrhea. Hypomagnesemia should be ruled out.

- The transtubular potassium gradient may be useful to differentiate types of renal K^+ loss. It is calculated as follows:

$$TTKG = \frac{U[K^+]}{P[K^+]} \div \frac{U_{osm}}{P_{osm}}$$

Calculation assumes Uosm >Posm.
TTKG <2 suggests renal loss due to increased distal flow; TTKG >4 suggests increased distal K+ secretion (see Fig. 16-3).

Evaluation

See Figure 16-3.

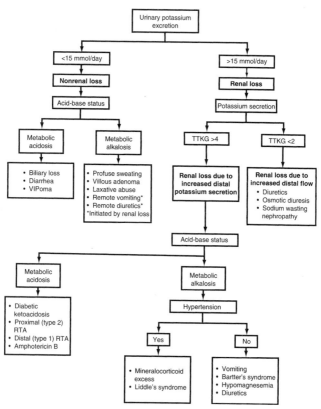

FIGURE 16-3. Evaluation of hypokalemia. TTKG, transtubular potassium gradient.

Treatment

- K^+ may be repleted either orally or intravenously. It is difficult to provide an algorithmic approach to replacing K^+ as the degree of depletion does not correlate well with plasma levels.

- It is generally safer and more cost effective to replace K^+ via the oral route. Caution should be used in replacing K^+ in patients with renal insufficiency. A reasonable estimate is that every 10 mEq of KCl will increase the serum level 0.05–0.1 mEq/L.

- Severe hypokalemia or patients who cannot take anything PO should be treated with IV KCl. The rate of infusion should not exceed 20 mmol/hr.

- If hypomagnesemia is present, magnesium oxide, 400 mg PO bid–tid should be given as well.

Hyperkalemia

… So much Kayexalate, so little time …

- Defined as a [K^+] in excess of 5 mmol/L, the most serious effect is cardiac toxicity. If a suspicious result is received, consider repeating it stat; a potassium can be obtained on an ABG. An ECG must be obtained. Refer to ECG interpretation section later in this chapter. Look for peaked T waves, prolonged PR interval, and QRS duration. Consider continuous cardiac monitoring if the potassium is >6.5.

Etiology

- **Pseudohyperkalemia** is caused by K^+ movement out of cells associated with venipuncture. This may be seen with repeated fist clenching, prolonged tourniquet time, hemolysis, leukocytosis, or thrombocytosis.

- **Increased K^+ intake** is an unusual cause of hyperkalemia but may be seen with excess K^+ replacement, renal insufficiency, or both.

- **Transcellular shifts** of K^+ may cause hyperkalemia. This may be seen with acidosis, insulin deficiency, drugs (succinylcholine, β- blockers), hypertonicity (e.g., hyperglycemia), hemolysis, tumor lysis, rhabdomyolysis, and hyperkalemic periodic paralysis.

- **Decreased renal K^+ excretion** is the usual cause of chronic hyperkalemia.

Major Causes of Decreased Renal Potassium Excretion

- Renal failure

- Volume depletion

- Primary hypoaldosteronism

- Secondary hypoaldosteronism (e.g., diabetes, mild renal failure, chronic tubulointerstitial disease)

- Drugs (e.g., nonsteroidal antiinflammatory drugs, ACE inhibitor, angiotensin receptor blockers, heparin, spironolactone, triamterene, amiloride, trimethoprim, pentamidine)

- Tubulointerstitial disease (e.g., systemic lupus erythematosus, sickle cell disease, multiple myeloma)

- Type 4 renal tubular acidosis

Evaluation

- Rule out pseudohyperkalemia by repeating the serum electrolytes. Consider drawing the sample without the use of a tourniquet or fist clenching.

- If the patient has thrombocytosis or marked leukocytosis, the sample may be drawn in a heparinized tube.

- Obtain a stat ECG and an ABG (if acidosis is a concern).

- Assess the patient's urine output and renal function.

- Examine the patient, paying particular attention to ECF volume status.

- Review the patient's medication list.

- Determination of plasma renin and aldosterone levels may be useful.

Treatment

- Stop all exogenous K^+ and potentially offending drugs.

- Severe hyperkalemia or hyperkalemia with ECG changes requires emergent treatment. **Do not do this by yourself.** Call your resident immediately.

- **Acute treatment**

  - **Calcium gluconate** 10%, 10 mL IV over 2–3 minutes decreases cardiac membrane excitability. The effect occurs in minutes but lasts only 30–60 minutes. It can be repeated after 5–10 minutes if the ECG does not change. Use with extreme caution in patients receiving digoxin.

  - **Insulin**, 10–20 units IV, causes an intracellular shift of K^+ in 10–30 minutes. The effect lasts for several hours. **Glucose**, 50 gms IV (1 amp D50), should also be administered to prevent hypoglycemia.

  - **NaHCO₃**, 1 ampule IV can also be used to cause an intracellular shift of K^+, and the effect can last several hours. This treatment should probably be reserved for patients with severe hyperkalemia and metabolic acidosis. Patients with end-stage renal disease seldom respond and may not tolerate the Na^+ load.

  - **β_2-Adrenergic agonists** can be used to cause an intracellular shift of K^+.

  - **Diuretics** (e.g., furosemide, 40–120 mg IV) enhance K^+ excretion provided renal function is adequate.

  - **Cation exchange resins** (sodium polystyrene sulfonate, Kayexalate) enhance K^+ excretion from the GI tract. Kayexalate may be given PO (20–50 g in 100–200 mL 20% sorbitol) or as a retention enema (50 g in 200 mL 20% sorbitol). The effect may not be evident for several hours and lasts 4–6 hours. Doses may be repeated every 4–6 hours as needed.

- **Dialysis** may be necessary for severe hyperkalemia when other measures are ineffective and for patients with renal failure.

- **Chronic treatment** is aimed at the underlying condition. Dietary K^+ should be restricted. Metabolic acidosis should be corrected. Drugs causing hyperkalemia should be avoided. Administration of exogenous mineralocorticoid may be effective for select patients.

VITAL SIGNS

… Occupational hazard: pager-induced intern tachycardia and tachypnea …

Although it often seems that the nursing personnel are much more concerned about alterations in vital signs than the physicians, you should take all such calls seriously. If the nurse seems really concerned, you should just go see the patient and assess the situation for yourself.

Blood Pressure

- You will frequently be called with high and low BPs. Be sure you know what the patient's baseline BP has been and recheck the BP yourself before rendering a judgment.

- It is also important to know if the patient is taking any antihypertensive drugs and if they have been given recently.

- **Marked hypotension** should be dealt with emergently. Go see the patient immediately; do not attempt to handle this by phone. Be sure to recheck the BP yourself and assess the other vital signs. The evaluation and management of hypotension is discussed in Chapter 12. Above all, if you find that you're in over your head, call your resident immediately.

- You will often be called regarding **relative hypotension** and whether certain medications should be given (e.g., β-blockers, ACE inhibitors, calcium channel blockers, diuretics). As a general rule, if the patient is asymptomatic and the medications necessary (e.g., for congestive heart failure), the medications may be given. If multiple medications are to be given, consider giving some now and some later.

- Calls for high BP are annoyingly frequent. Resist the temptation to treat **modest elevations**. This is particularly true in patients with a recent stroke.

- Patients with **marked elevations** of BP should be seen immediately. Recheck the BP yourself (be sure the cuff is large enough for the patient's arm) in both arms. Evaluation and management of hypertension are discussed further in Chapter 12.

- Alternatively, if the patient is already taking an antihypertensive agent, consider giving an additional dose or the next dose early.

Heart Rate

- An ECG should be done in all with bradycardia or tachycardia. Tachyarrhythmias and bradyarrhythmias are discussed in detail in the ECG Interpretation section, later in this chapter.

- Nursing may wish to hold β-blockers and calcium channel blockers in the setting of relative bradycardia. If the patient is asymptomatic and the heart rate at least 60, they can usually be given. You may consider reducing the dose or giving the medications at different times.

Respiratory Rate

- **Tachypnea** should always be taken seriously; it is a *must see*. It is almost always associated with shortness of breath, which is discussed in Chapter 12.

- A markedly **reduced respiratory rate** is equally serious. Again be sure to measure it yourself (count for a full minute).

- Observe the respiratory pattern closely. Is there a Cheyne-Stokes pattern, which can drastically alter the respiratory rate? Was the patient asleep when the low respiratory rate was recorded? What is the patient's mental status now? Is the patient's airway open and secure? Is the patient taking sedative medications (e.g., narcotics)?

- Checking the O_2 saturation is a good idea, but it tells you nothing about the alveolar ventilation (P_{CO_2}). An ABG is much more informative—if you're considering it, you probably should go ahead and get it!

Temperature

- Fever is one of the most common calls an intern receives. Why does it seem this always happens at 4:00 PM or 4:00 AM? (*But don't lose your cool....*)

- The evaluation and management of fever are discussed in Chapter 12.

ELECTROCARDIOGRAPHIC INTERPRETATION

... NSR, no abnormalities—an intern's dream ...

This section assumes a basic understanding of ECG reading and does not review the fundamentals.

Narrow Complex Tachycardias

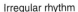

Narrow complex tachycardia

Irregular rhythm
- Atrial fibrillation
- Multifocal atrial tachycardia

Regular rhythm
- Sinus tachycardia
- AV node reentrant tachycardia
- Atrial flutter

Sinus Tachycardia

Key Features
- The P wave is of the usual morphology and rates range from 100–160 bpm.

- The QRS maintains its baseline appearance, but rate-related aberrancy occasionally occurs.

- It does not develop or resolve in a paroxysmal fashion.

- Differential diagnosis includes pain, fever, hypovolemia, hyperthyroidism, pulmonary embolism, anxiety, and ischemia.

Management
- Treatment is aimed at the underlying cause.

Atrioventricular Nodal Reentrant Tachycardia

Key Features
- Probably the most common cause of paroxysmal regular SVT.

- Requires two physiologically distinct pathways of conduction (one fast and one slow) in the AV node.

- During NSR, conduction through the AV node occurs over the fast pathway.

- The rate is usually between 150 and 250 bpm.

- The QRS is usually narrow but can be widened because of a preexisting conduction delay (e.g., BBB) or rate-related aberrancy.

- In **common (typical or slow-fast) AVNRT,** there is antegrade conduction over the slow pathway and retrograde conduction back to the atria over the fast pathway, completing the reentrant circuit. Negative P waves are usually buried in the QRS but may rarely be seen in II, III, and aVF. It is usually initiated by an APC.

- In the much more **uncommon** (**atypical or fast-slow**) **AVNRT** the circuit is reversed. Negative P waves are usually seen in II, III, and aVF. It is usually initiated by a VPC.

Management

- Initial treatment of acute episodes in hemodynamically stable patients begins with vagal maneuvers (e.g., Valsalva's, carotid massage).

- If this is unsuccessful, adenosine (6 mg IV followed by 12 mg IV if necessary—halve dosage if giving via central line) should be tried.

- Patients who are hemodynamically unstable should be electrically cardioverted.

Preexcitation Syndromes

Key Features

- Requires the presence of an accessory pathway.

- Approximately one-fourth of accessory pathways are concealed and conduct in a retrograde fashion only.

- When the accessory pathway is able to conduct in an antegrade manner during SR, pre-excitation (early activation of the ventricles) occurs. This results in a short PR and a delta wave (initial slurring of the QRS), the Wolff-Parkinson-White syndrome (WPW) (Fig. 16-4).

- During **orthodromic AVRT** conduction is antegrade through the AV node and His-Purkinje system and retrograde through the accessory pathway, completing the reentrant circuit. It may occur with a concealed pathway or in WPW. Rates range from 150–250 bpm. The QRS can maintain its baseline appearance but may also show rate-related aberrancy. Inverted P waves may be seen at the end of the QRS complex. It is paroxysmal, often initiated by an APC or VPC.

- Patients with WPW can also have an **antidromic AVRT** in which conduction in the reentrant circuit is reversed (antegrade through the

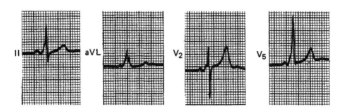

FIGURE 16-4. Wolff-Parkinson-White syndrome with preexcitation.

accessory pathway and retrograde through the AV node and His-Purkinje system). The QRS is also wide in this instance, but this is actually less common than WPW with orthodromic AVRT and aberrant conduction.

- AF and atrial flutter in patients with WPW can be serious because of fast conduction rates and the propensity to initiate VF.

Management

- Narrow complex orthodromic AVRT can be treated the same as AVNRT.

- Treatment of wide complex tachycardias requires careful consideration. Unless it is orthodromic AVRT with aberrancy (which can be impossible to determine based on a surface ECG), **treatment with drugs that slow AV conduction (i.e., adenosine, beta-blockers, calcium-channel blockers, digoxin) may actually increase the ventricular rate with disastrous consequences**. When hemodynamically stable, IV procainamide or amiodarone should be used. If you don't know what you're dealing with (and you probably won't), **get help as soon as possible**. If hemodynamically unstable, the patient should be electrically cardioverted.

Atrial Tachycardia

Key Features

- A single different P-wave morphology is seen in **unifocal atrial tachycardia**. Rate is usually between 100 and 200 bpm. The QRS usually maintains its baseline appearance but aberrancy can occur. It is a less common cause of SVT.

- In **multifocal atrial tachycardia** (**MAT**) there are at least three separate P-wave morphologies; the rate is over 100 bpm and irregular. There is variation in the PR interval. It is most often seen in acutely ill elderly patients with pulmonary disease or CHF.

Management

- When not associated with digitalis toxicity, unifocal atrial tachycardia may be treated with calcium channel blockers or β-blockers.

- Treatment of MAT is focused on the underlying condition.

Atrial Fibrillation

Key Features

- Atrial activity is completely disorganized. The baseline is wavy without clear P waves (Fig. 16-5).

- The ventricular rate is irregularly irregular and may be slow to fast (usually >100 bpm in untreated patients).

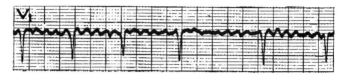

FIGURE 16-5. Atrial fibrillation.

- The QRS typically maintains its usual morphology. Variable rate-related aberrancy may also be seen.

- The incidence of AF increases with age and there are many possible causes including CAD, MI, valvular disease, PE, COPD, pericarditis, hyperthyroidism, acute alcohol intoxication, and idiopathic.

Management

- If the patient is unstable (infarction, ischemia, hypotension, mental status alteration), immediate electrical cardioversion is indicated.

- When the patient is stable, rate control may be achieved with AV nodal blocking agents:

  - Diltiazem, 0.25 mg/kg IVP over 2 minutes; if no response, repeat 0.35 mg/kg IVP over 2 minutes; follow with an IV infusion at 5–15 mg/hr. Diltiazem is probably the agent of choice in most patients. Verapamil, 5–15 mg IVP then continuous infusion at 0.05–0.2 mg/min, can also be used.

  - Metoprolol, 5 mg IVP every 5 minutes to a total of 15 mg followed by oral dosing. Preferred agent if ischemia is suspected or present.

  - Digoxin, 0.25–0.5 mg IVP; then 0.125–0.25 mg IVP every 4–6 hours to a total dose of 0.75–1.35 mg; followed by oral dosing. Digoxin's effect will take longer than other agents.

  - Amiodarone, 150 mg IV over 10 minutes, followed by infusion of 1 mg/min for 6 hours, then 0.5 mg/min for 18 hours, is not FDA-approved for treatment of atrial fibrillation, but studies have shown it to be effective. Its onset of action is slower than calcium channel blockers and beta-blockers. Also, be cautious if atrial fibrillation has been present >48 hours as amiodarone can cause conversion to sinus rhythm and put the patient at risk for cardioembolic stroke.

  - If the patient has an EF <40% or CHF, amiodarone and digoxin are the preferred agents.

- Pharmacotherapy for AF with WPW and pre-excitation is of special concern (see previous discussion).

- In stable patients, anticoagulation is generally recommended before cardioversion (chemical or electrical) if AF has been present for >48 hours or the duration is unknown.

Atrial Flutter

Key Features

- Atrial flutter is characterized by flutter waves in a regular, undulating, sawtooth pattern at a rate of 280–350 bpm. Flutter waves are best seen in leads II, III, aVF, and V_1 (Fig. 16-6).

- The ventricular rate depends on the degree of AV block (2:1, 3:1) and may be regular or variable.

- Vagal maneuvers or adenosine may slow AV conduction, revealing the flutter waves.

- The QRS maintains its baseline appearance.

- Atrial flutter is most commonly seen in those conditions associated with AF (see previous discussion).

Management

- Management of atrial flutter is similar to that for AF.

- Patients who are unstable should be immediately electrically cardioverted.

- Rate control in stable patients may be achieved in a similar manner as for AF.

Wide Complex Tachycardias

Wide complex tachycardias may be of either supraventricular or ventricular origin. Differentiation of SVT with aberrant conduction from VT on the basis of the surface ECG may be difficult (if not impossible in some patients). This differentiation is not merely academic but critical to appropriate treatment. If you find yourself in this predicament,

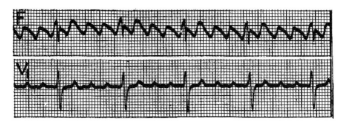

FIGURE 16-6. Atrial flutter.

call for help immediately. Regardless of the cause, if the patient is unstable (ischemia or infarction, hypotension, CHF, altered mental status), electrical cardioversion is indicated.

Ventricular Tachycardia

... This is bad. Really bad. Call for backup now ...

Key Features

- VT is the most frequent life-threatening arrhythmia, and it is most often associated with MI.

- VT is defined as more than three ventricular complexes in a row at a rate of 100–250. Sustained VT lasts longer than 30 seconds or is associated with hemodynamic collapse.

- The QRS is >120 milliseconds and often has an LBBB pattern. The T wave is usually in the opposite direction of the main QRS deflection (Fig. 16-7). It may be monomorphic (single QRS morphology) or polymorphic (multiple QRS morphologies).

- AV dissociation is present but usually cannot be easily seen.

- There may be occasional capture, fusion beats, or both.

- VT is often associated with hemodynamic compromise and has a distressing tendency to degenerate into VF and death.

- VT can easily be confused with SVT with rate-related aberrancy or a pre-existent intraventricular conduction defect, antidromic AVRT, and pre-excited AF (see previous discussion).

Management

- If a wide complex tachycardia cannot be immediately and definitively diagnosed, it should initially be treated as VT, and you should call for help at once!

- Sustained VT (or any other wide complex tachycardia) in unstable patients requires immediate DC cardioversion by ACLS protocol.

- Pharmacologic treatment may be attempted in stable VT patients using amiodarone, lidocaine, or procainamide. See ACLS algorithm, Chapter 2. Of course, you'll call for help before you do this!

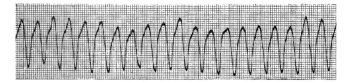

FIGURE 16-7. Ventricular tachycardia.

Torsades de Pointes

Key Features

- TDP is a rapid, polymorphic VT with QRS complexes that oscillate in amplitude and morphology, producing the appearance of a continuously twisting axis of depolarization.

- It is usually preceded by a prolonged QT interval and initiated by a VPC.

- It may be associated with electrolyte-induced long QT (most notably hypokalemia and hypomagnesemia), drugs that prolong the QT, congenital long QT syndromes, and end-stage cardiomyopathy.

- It often occurs for brief periods but can be sustained with hemodynamic collapse.

Management

- Sustained, unstable TDP should be treated with electrical cardioversion.

- Offending drugs should be stopped, and electrolyte abnormalities should be corrected.

- IV magnesium sulfate 1–2 g (up to 4–6 g) can be highly effective, even if the magnesium level is normal.

Ventricular Fibrillation

… Close this book immediately! There should be multiple people running toward the patient with powerful electrical equipment …

Key Features

- VF is characterized by completely chaotic, rapid, highly variable amplitude electrical activity emanating from the ventricles. There are no discernible QRS complexes.

- There is no effective cardiac output, and if VF remains untreated, it rapidly results in death.

Management

- All patients require immediate electrical cardioversion by ACLS protocol.

Conduction Abnormalities

First-Degree Atrioventricular Block

Key Features

- The PR interval is lengthened (>200 milliseconds), but all P waves are conducted to the ventricles (Fig. 16-8).

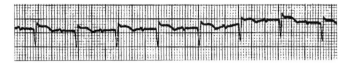

FIGURE 16-8. First-degree AV block.

- It is associated with increased vagal tone, conduction system degeneration, ischemia, drugs (e.g., antiarrhythmics, calcium channel blockers, β-blockers), and electrolyte abnormalities.

Management
- Primary AV block is almost always asymptomatic and rarely requires any specific treatment.

Second-Degree Atrioventricular Block, Mobitz Type I (*Wenckebach's Disease*)

Key Features
- Not all of the atrial impulses are conducted.

- There is a progressive delay in AV conduction before a completely blocked P wave. This results in a progressive prolongation of the PR interval and shortening of the RR interval before a nonconducted P wave (Fig. 16-9).

- The QRS complexes maintain their baseline appearance and appear in regular groupings. This grouping should immediately raise suspicion for Mobitz type I second-degree AV block.

- The site of conduction block is almost always within the AV node.

- Etiologies are the same as for primary AV block. Ischemia, particularly in the inferior or posterior distribution, is a common cause.

- It is usually benign and generally does not degenerate to complete heart block.

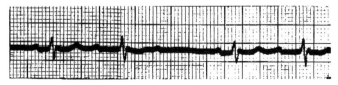

FIGURE 16-9. Mobitz type I (Wenckebach), second-degree AV block.

Management

- Mobitz type I second-degree AV block is usually asymptomatic and transient. Treatment is generally not necessary unless the patient is symptomatic.

- If symptomatic, atropine (0.5–1 mg IV repeated every 3–5 minutes prn to a total dose of 0.04 mg/kg) may be given, and if persistent, cardiac pacing may be necessary.

Second-Degree Atrioventricular Block, Mobitz Type II

Key Features

- Not all of the atrial impulses are conducted; however, there is no preceding conduction block.

- The PR interval is fixed and usually normal with suddenly and intermittently blocked P waves (Fig. 16-10).

- Blocked conduction may occur at a fixed ratio (e.g., 2:1, 3:1, 4:1).

- The site of conduction block is usually infranodal within the His-Purkinje system.

- Causes include increased vagal tone, conduction system disease, antiarrhythmic drugs, and ischemia (particularly in the anterior distribution).

- Mobitz type II second-degree AV block usually implies severe conduction system disease and often precedes the development of complete heart block, especially when a bundle branch block is also present. Therefore, you should always take this rhythm very seriously.

Management

- Symptomatic patients should initially be treated with atropine (0.5–1 mg IV repeated every 3–5 minutes prn to a total dose of 0.04 mg/kg), but the response is typically poor and temporary.

- Pacemaker placement is frequently indicated, regardless of whether the patient is symptomatic.

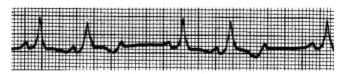

FIGURE 16-10. Mobitz type II, second-degree AV block.

Third-Degree (Complete) Atrioventricular Block

Key Features

- As the name implies, AV block is complete, and no P waves are conducted to the ventricles (Fig. 16-11).

- An automatic focus below the block takes over at its own intrinsic rate (usually slower than the P wave rate, <50).

- There is no fixed relationship between the P waves and the QRS complexes (AV dissociation).

- The QRS complexes are usually wide but may be narrow if they arise from a junctional focus.

- The site of conduction block may be AV node or more typically within the His-Purkinje system.

- Third-degree AV block may be congenital or acquired. Etiologies of acquired complete heart block include idiopathic conduction system degeneration, ischemia or infarct, infiltrative diseases, drug toxicity, calcific aortic stenosis, endocarditis, and cardiac surgery.

Management

- Emergent treatment with atropine (0.5–1 mg IV repeated every 3–5 minutes prn to a total dose of 0.04 mg/kg), and pacemaker placement is usually required.

Myocardial Ischemia and Infarction

Key Features

- Myocardial ischemia is characterized by symmetric T-wave inversion that may be slight to deep, flat or down-sloping ST depression, or both.

- The ECG typically demonstrates sequential changes during the evolution of an acute ST-elevation MI (Fig. 16–12). Certainly not all patients show this typical sequence, and the time course of the changes may vary among patients.

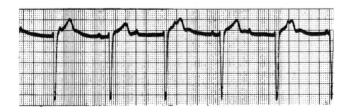

FIGURE 16-11. Complete heart block.

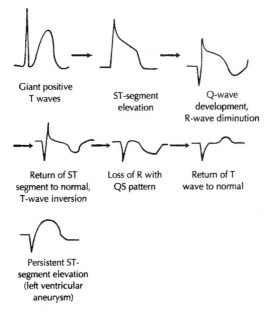

FIGURE 16-12. ST and T-wave changes in MI. (From Alpert J. *Cardiology for the primary care physician.* Appleton and Lange, 1998: 168, with permission.)

- In the earliest hyperacute phase tall and prolonged T waves are seen.

- This is followed by the acute phase of convex-up ST-segment elevation in the leads facing the area of injury.

- Reciprocal ST depression may be seen in the leads opposite to the area of infarction.

- Over the following hours to days, the R-wave amplitude decreases and pathologic Q waves appear (>40 milliseconds or greater than or equal to one-third of the entire QRS amplitude).

- As the ST segments return to baseline, the T waves become symmetrically inverted.

- Over time, the T waves may return to their baseline orientation.

- The distribution of these typical ECG changes can be used to predict the location of the myocardial infarction (Table 16-1). It is important to remember, however, that this method of localization can be rather imprecise.

TABLE 16-1.
ELECTROCARDIOGRAPHIC LOCALIZATION OF
MYOCARDIAL INFARCTION

Area of MI	ECG abnormality	Artery involved
Septal	ST elevation and Q waves V_1–V_2	Proximal left anterior descending, septal perforators
Anteroseptal	ST elevation and Q waves V_1–V_4	Left anterior descending
Anterior	ST elevation and Q waves V_3–V_4	Left anterior descending
Anterolateral	ST elevation and Q waves I, aVL, V_3–V_6	Mid-left anterior descending or circumflex
Extensive anterior	ST elevation and Q waves I, aVL, V_1–V_6	Proximal left anterior descending
Lateral	ST elevation and Q waves I, aVL, V_6	Circumflex
High lateral	ST elevation and Q waves I, aVL	Circumflex
Inferior	ST elevation and Q waves II, III, aVF	Right coronary artery
Posterior	Tall R and ST depression V_1–V_2	Right coronary artery or circumflex
Right ventricular	ST elevation V_4R	Proximal right coronary artery

- The ST segments may remain chronically elevated in the setting of LV aneurysm formation.

- Noninfarction-related Q waves can be seen in myocarditis, cardiomyopathies, muscular dystrophies, scleroderma, amyloidosis, sarcoidosis, WPW, LVH, BBB, COPD, and PE.

- Non-ST elevation MIs often have much more nonspecific and subtle ECG changes. Possible changes include persistent ST depression, T-wave inversions, loss of QRS amplitude, and poor R-wave progression across the precordium.

- Prior MIs and preexistent or newly developed conduction abnormalities may mask or make these typical changes difficult to interpret.

- Other conditions may mimic the ECG changes of an acute MI including pericarditis, myocarditis, and aortic dissection.

- It is very difficult to diagnose acute MI changes in the setting of LBBB or a paced rhythm.

Management

- A detailed discussion of the management of myocardial ischemia and infarction is beyond the scope of this manual. Refer to the Chapter 12 section on chest pain for acute management and call your resident immediately.

Miscellaneous Conditions
Pericarditis

Key Features

- The acute phase of pericarditis is characterized by diffuse flat or concave-up ST-segment elevation, particularly in the precordial leads. The entire T wave may be lifted off the baseline, and there may also be diffuse PR depression (Fig. 16-13).

- In the intermediate phase, diffuse T-wave inversion appears and ST elevation resolves.

- In the late phase, T-wave inversion resolves.

- There is no development of Q waves.

- Pericarditis has many possible causes including infectious (viral, bacterial, fungal, tuberculous), post-MI, posttraumatic, postpericardiotomy, collagen vascular diseases, drug-induced (hydralazine, procainamide), uremia, infiltrative (sarcoidosis, amyloidosis), neoplastic, radiation, and idiopathic.

Management

- Specific, treatable causes should be managed in the appropriate manner (e.g., antimicrobial agents for infectious causes or dialysis for uremia).

- Antiinflammatory treatment may be effective (NSAIDs or prednisone).

- Narcotic analgesics may be given for refractory pain.

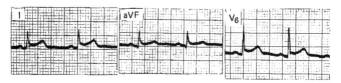

FIGURE 16-13. Pericarditis.

- Patients should be observed closely for the development of cardiac tamponade.

- Anticoagulants should be avoided because of the risk of hemopericardium.

Hyperkalemia

Key Features

- The earliest ECG feature of hyperkalemia is tall, peaked, symmetric, narrow-based T waves. These are often referred to as "tented" T waves. They are best seen in leads II, III, and V_2-V_4 (Fig. 16-14).

- The P-wave amplitude then decreases and the PR interval becomes prolonged. With increasingly severe hyperkalemia, the P waves eventually all but disappear. Consequently, arrhythmias that are common in hyperkalemia can be difficult to identify.

- With severe hyperkalemia, the QRS progressively widens, the R amplitude decreases, and S waves become prominent. There may also be ST-segment depression or elevation.

- Eventually, with extreme hyperkalemia, the ECG takes on a slow sinusoidal pattern that may degenerate into asystole or VF if not immediately and aggressively treated.

Management

- The acute management of hyperkalemia is covered in the section regarding electrolyte abnormalities, earlier in this chapter.

Digitalis Effect and Toxicity

Key Features

- At therapeutic levels, digitalis may cause a characteristic, gradual down-sloping, concave-up (also described as "scooping" or "sagging") of the ST segment. The ST is typically depressed and shortened and the T wave amplitude decreased. Collectively, this is known as the "dig effect" (Fig. 16-15).

- At times, it can be difficult to differentiate the dig effect from other causes of ST depression.

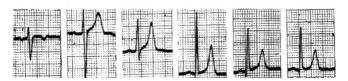

FIGURE 16-14. Hyperkalemia.

- Digitalis toxicity has been associated with nearly all known arrhythmias. Common digitalis toxicity associated arrhythmias include sinus block, APCs, PAT with block, JPCs, junctional tachycardia, AV block, VPCs, VT (including bidirectional VT), and VF.

- Hypokalemia, hypomagnesemia, and hypercalcemia may enhance the toxic effects of digitalis.

- Because of its narrow therapeutic window, toxicity can occur even when the digitalis level is within the usual therapeutic range.

Management

- Digitalis should be discontinued immediately.

- In the setting of recent acute ingestion of potentially toxic amounts of digitalis and before toxic cardiac side effects have occurred, induced emesis or gastric lavage may be used. Activated charcoal may also be administered to reduce further absorption.

- The patient should be on continuous telemetry monitoring.

- Electrolyte abnormalities (particularly hypokalemia) should be carefully corrected. However, care should be taken as rapid increases in potassium (even within the normal range) may worsen AV conduction and lead to complete heart block. Serum potassium concentration should be determined before potassium administration. Massive digitalis overdoses can cause hyperkalemia.

- Ventricular arrhythmias can be treated with IV lidocaine (1–1.5 mg/kg initial IV bolus, additional 0.5–1.5 mg/kg IV bolus injections prn up to a total of 3 mg/kg, followed by continuous IV infusion at 2–4 mg/minute) or phenytoin (250 mg IV loading dose over 10 minutes, followed by additional 100 mg IV doses every 5 minutes prn to a total of 1,000 mg). Avoid procainamide and bretylium.

- Bradyarrhythmias may be treated with atropine (0.5–1 mg IV repeated every 3–5 minutes prn to a total dose of 0.04 mg/kg) or temporary pacing.

- Digitalis-specific Fab antibody fragments (Digibind) may be given when other methods have been ineffective. One vial of Fab fragments is equivalent to 40 mg and neutralizes approximately 0.6 mg of

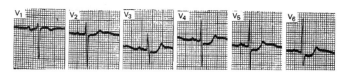

FIGURE 16-15. Digitalis effect.

digitalis. The dosage for chronic toxicity is calculated as follows: Number of vials = [dig level (ng/mL) × weight (kg)]/100. For acute overdosages, use the following formula: Number of vials = [total amount ingested (mg) × 0.8]/0.5. If acute ingestion and unknown dosage, give 10–20 vials IV. The Fab fragments are given in NS over 15–30 minutes.

- Electrical cardioversion should be used only as a last resort, when all other measures have failed. Cardioversion in the setting of digitalis toxicity can cause VT or VF that is resistant to any further cardioversion.

ACID–BASE DISORDERS

... Retention, compensation, deficits ...

- Changes in acid–base balance occur as a result of changes in $[H^+]$ and $[HCO_3^-]$.

- **Acidemia** results from either decreased $[HCO_3^-]$ or increased P_{CO_2}.

- **Alkalemia** results from either increased $[HCO_3^-]$ or decreased P_{CO_2}.

- An ABG and a serum $[HCO_3^-]$ are required to assess acid/base status

- Stepwise approach to an ABG:

  1. Examine the pH. Is the patient acidemic or alkalemic?

  2. Examine the $[HCO_3^-]$. In primary metabolic disorders, it moves in the same direction as the pH.

  3. Examine the P_{CO_2}. In primary respiratory disorders, it moves in the opposite direction as the pH.

  4. Is there adequate respiratory or metabolic compensation? If there is not adequate compensation, there may be a mixed disorder present. (Table 16-2.)

  5. If a metabolic acidosis is present, calculate the anion gap. If no gap is present, calculate the urine anion gap.

  See the diagram on the inside back cover of this book.

Metabolic Acidosis
Etiology
See Table 16-3.

Treatment
- Treatment of the underlying condition should be the primary focus.

- Severe acidosis (pH <7.20) may require treatment with parenteral NaHCO3. Rapid infusion should be considered only for severe acidosis.

TABLE 16-2.
PRIMARY ACID–BASE DISORDERS

Disorder	Abnormality	Primary changes	Compensatory response
Metabolic acidosis	$[HCO_3^-]$ loss or $[H^+]$ gain	$\downarrow[HCO_3^-]$	$\downarrow$$P_{CO_2}$ by 1.0–1.3 mm Hg for every 1.0 mmol/L $\downarrow[HCO_3^-]$
Metabolic alkalosis	$[H^+]$ loss or $[HCO_3^-]$ gain	$\uparrow[HCO_3^-]$	$\uparrow$$P_{CO_2}$ 0.6–0.7 mm Hg for every 1 mmol/L $\uparrow[HCO_3^-]$
Respiratory acidosis	Alveolar hypoventilation	$\uparrow$$P_{CO_2}$	
Acute			$\uparrow[HCO_3^-]$ 1.0 mmol/L for every 10 mm Hg $\uparrow$$P_{CO_2}$
Chronic			$\uparrow[HCO_3^-]$ 3.0–3.5 mmol/L for every 10 mm Hg $\uparrow$$P_{CO_2}$
Respiratory alkalosis	Alveolar hyper-ventilation	$\downarrow$$P_{CO_2}$	
Acute			$\downarrow[HCO_3^-]$ 2.0 mmol/L for every 10 mm Hg $\downarrow$$P_{CO_2}$
Chronic			$\downarrow[HCO_3^-]$ 4.0–5.0 mmol/L for every 10 mm Hg $\downarrow$$P_{CO_2}$

See the diagram on the inside back cover of this book.

- The bicarbonate deficit may be calculated as follows:
- $[HCO_3^-]$ deficit (mEq/L) = $[0.5 \times$ body wt (kg)$]$ − $(24$ − measured $[HCO_3^-])$

- Overaggressive correction should be avoided to prevent overshoot alkalosis.
- Hypernatremia and fluid overload can occur with $NaHCO_3$ administration.
- Serum electrolytes should be followed closely.

Metabolic Alkalosis
Etiology
- Metabolic alkalosis may be caused by HCO_3^- gain/H^+ loss or volume contraction.

TABLE 16-3.
CAUSES OF METABOLIC ACIDOSIS

Increased anion gap	Normal anion gap
Uremia	GI [HCO_3^-] loss (diarrhea, urinary diversion, small bowel, biliary, pancreatic, cholestyramine, or ingestion of Ca or Mg chloride)
Diabetic ketoacidosis; alcoholic ketoacidosis	Ingestion of exogenous acids
Lactic acidosis	Proximal (type 2) renal tubular acidosis
Methanol	Classic distal (type 1) renal tubular acidosis
Paraldehyde	Hyperkalemic (type 4) renal tubular acidosis
Ethylene glycol	Early renal insufficiency
Salicylates	Expansion acidosis (rapid saline administration)
	Drug-induced hyperkalemia (K^+-sparing diuretics, trimethoprim, pentamidine, ACE inhibitors, nonsteroidal antiinflammatory drugs, cyclosporine), carbonic anhydrase inhibitors

- Vomiting and diuretic use are the two most common causes.

- See Table 16-4.

Treatment

- Treatment of the underlying condition should be the primary focus.

- When volume contraction is present, it should be corrected with isotonic NS.

- Hypokalemia and hypomagnesemia should be corrected.

- Cl unresponsive causes do not improve with administration of NaCl; in fact, it may be hazardous.

- K^+ sparing diuretics may be effective for some forms of hyperaldosteronism.

Respiratory Acidosis
Etiology

- ↑P_{CO_2} is almost always the result of alveolar hypoventilation.

- In **acute respiratory acidosis,** the pH ↓0.08 for every 10 mm Hg ↑P_{CO_2} above 40.

TABLE 16-4.
CAUSES OF METABOLIC ALKALOSIS

Cl⁻ Responsive (Urine Cl⁻ <10 mmol/L)	Cl⁻ Unresponsive (Urine Cl⁻ >10 mmol/L)
Gastrointestinal	Normotensive
Vomiting, NG suction	K^+ or Mg^{2+} depletion
Villous adenoma	Bartter's syndrome
Congenital chloridorrhea	Hypercalcemia
Cystic fibrosis	Hypertensive
Renal	Primary aldosteronism
Diuretics	Hyperreninemic hyperaldosteronism
Posthypercapnic state	Adrenal enzyme defects
Nonreabsorbable anions (penicillin)	Cushing's syndrome
Exogenous alkali ($NaHCO_3^-$ massive transfusion, antacids, acetate, citrate)	Exogenous mineralocorticoid
Contraction alkalosis	Pseudohyperaldosteronism (licorice, carbenoxolone, tobacco chewing, Liddle's syndrome)

- In **chronic respiratory acidosis,** the pH ↓0.03 for every 10 mm Hg ↑P_{CO_2} above 40.
- Renal compensation takes several days to develop fully.
- See Table 16-5.

TABLE 16-5.
CAUSES OF RESPIRATORY ACIDOSIS

Central respiratory depression (drugs, sleep apnea, obesity, CNS disease)

Airway obstruction (foreign body, laryngospasm, severe bronchospasm)

Neuromuscular abnormalities (polio, kyphoscoliosis, myasthenia, muscular dystrophy)

Parenchymal lung disease (COPD, pneumothorax, pneumonia, pulmonary edema, interstitial lung disease)

Treatment

- Treatment is directed at the underlying condition.

- Potentially contributing drugs should be stopped or counteracted (e.g., naloxone, flumazenil).

- Ventilatory assistance may be required (CPAP or mechanical ventilation).

- Generally, $NaHCO_3$ treatment is not given, unless the patient is ventilated and the pH remains severely low.

Respiratory Alkalosis
Etiology

- It is important to remember that tachypnea/hyperventilation does not necessarily imply a simple respiratory alkalosis. If you have any uncertainty, obtain an ABG.

- See Table 16-6.

Treatment

- Treatment is directed at the underlying condition.

- Psychogenic hyperventilation may be treated by rebreathing from a paper bag.

TABLE 16-6.
CAUSES OF RESPIRATORY ALKALOSIS

Central stimulation (anxiety, pain, hyperventilation syndrome, head trauma, CVA, tumors, fever/infection, salicylates, thyroxine, progesterone)

Hypoxemia (any causes)

Airway irritation

Decreased lung compliance (CHF, fibrosis)

Pulmonary embolism

Hepatic insufficiency/failure

Pregnancy

Hyperthyroidism

Overzealous mechanical ventilation

RADIOGRAPH INTERPRETATION

... Know your patients inside out ...

Chest X-Ray

The chest x-ray is by far the most common radiograph you will order and need to interpret. When reading a chest x-ray, the most important thing is to be systematic. Be sure to check the name and date on the film and compare with old films whenever possible.

Technique

- Is the exposure correct? Underexposure can cause you to see things that aren't there, while overexposure can cause pathology to disappear. You should be able to faintly see the intervertebral spaces through the cardiac silhouette.

- Is the patient properly positioned? The spinous processes and trachea should be midline. The clavicular heads should be equidistant from the spinous processes. Rotated films distort the appearance of the cardiac silhouette and hila.

- Is the frontal film a PA or AP? AP films are often done in emergent situations or when the patient cannot stand. They can easily cause you to see things that aren't there.

- Was the film taken at full inspiration? If not, you may be seeing things again.

Airway

- The trachea should be midline and not deviated. The trachea will deviate towards the collapsed lung if there is a tension pneumothorax.

- If the patient is intubated, note the position of the endotracheal tube (should be about 2 cm above the carina).

Soft Tissues

- Examine the soft tissues for symmetry, subcutaneous air, edema, and breast tissue.

Bones

- Systematically look at the sternum, ribs, clavicles, spine, and shoulders.

- Look for fractures, osteolytic or osteoblastic lesions, and arthritic changes.

Diaphragm

- The sides of the diaphragm should be equal and slightly rounded. The right side may be slightly higher.

- Look for blunting of the costophrenic angles that suggest small pleural effusions.

- Flat diaphragms suggest emphysema.

- A unilateral high diaphragm may suggest paralysis, loss of lung volume on that side, or eventration.

- Check for free air under the diaphragm, which is an indication of perforation.

Heart and Mediastinum

- A maximal heart width greater than half of the chest width suggests cardiomegaly or pericardial effusion.

- The aortic knob should be distinct.

- Mediastinal widening is indicative of thoracic aortic dissection or aneurysm, pericardial effusion, or mass.

- Mediastinal and tracheal deviation may be seen with pneumothorax.

- Use lateral films to confirm findings on PA and look for retrocardiac infiltrates.

Hilar Structures

- The left hilum is usually 2–3 cm higher than the right. They are generally of equal size.

- Enlarged hila suggest lymphadenopathy.

Lung Fields

- Look for normal lung markings all the way out to the chest wall to rule out pneumothorax. Be sure not to miss this! If you think you've detected a pneumothorax, let your resident know right away.

- Normal lung markings taper as they travel out to the periphery and are smaller in the upper lungs. Lung markings in the upper lung fields that are as large or larger ("cephalization") suggest pulmonary edema.

- Kerley's B lines (small linear densities at the lateral lung bases) are also seen with CHF.

- Hyperlucency of the lung fields is seen in COPD.

- Examine the lung fields for the presence of infiltrates and masses.

- Obliteration of part or all of the heart border (silhouette sign) implies that the lesion is anterior. It may be located in the RML, lingula, or anterior segment of the upper lobe.

- A small pleural effusion is suggested by blunting of the costophrenic angle. Larger effusions obscure the shadow of the diaphragm and produce an upward-curving shadow along the chest wall. A straight horizontal fluid level indicates a concurrent pneumothorax.

- Lateral decubitus films should be done to ensure that the effusion is free flowing and large enough to attempt thoracentesis (usually >1 cm on lateral film).

Plain Abdominal Films

Generally speaking, plain abdominal films ("KUB" or "obstructive series") are of limited value. Despite that, they are ordered quite frequently. Again, a systematic approach is key.

Bones

- Examine the bones first or else you'll forget.

- Begin with the spine, then ribs, pelvis, and upper femurs. Look for signs of arthritis, fractures, and osteolytic or osteoblastic lesions.

Soft Tissues

- Systematically study the soft tissues looking for evidence of masses or calcifications.

- Be sure to carefully look for free air under the diaphragm (upright film) or next to the abdominal wall (lateral decubitus film). Free air is indicative of perforation. If you see this, let your resident know immediately!

Gastrointestinal Structures

- Look for the gastric bubble. A large air-distended stomach suggests some form of obstruction.

- Observe the bowel gas pattern. A small amount of air is generally seen in the colon, while the small bowel is generally devoid of air. Fecal material is often visible in the colon although large amounts may be seen in constipation.

- The colon may become greatly distended with air in colonic obstruction (colonic distention proximal to the obstruction) or ileus. Unless the distention is severe, the haustral markings are maintained. (The large bowel markings are differentiated from small bowel markings by their wider spacing, and the incomplete crossing of the lumen). When the ileocecal valve is incompetent, large bowel obstruction may also cause distention of the small bowel.

- Distention of the small bowel may be seen in mechanical obstruction and ileus. Small bowel striations are much more numerous and completely cross the lumen. With mechanical obstruction there is distention proximal to the obstruction and clearing of air distally.

- The appearance of ileus is much less distinct. There is discontinuous air in the small and usually large bowel. The degree of distention is also less remarkable and discontinuous.

- Air–fluid levels do not distinguish mechanical obstruction from ileus. They may be seen in both conditions.

PREPARATION FOR PROCEDURES

... A procedure canceled due to inadequate prep is like having a hemolyzed specimen. Nobody's happy, you have to do it again, and it's always the intern's fault ...

General Points

- Perform plain x-ray films prior to contrast studies. Perform contrast studies prior to barium studies (i.e., start with studies that require greatest amount of clarity of the area in question).

- Consult your radiology department if you have questions about what study to order or to confirm preparation for procedures. Some preparations are institution specific. See Table 16-7.

- Studies requiring no preparation include: chest x-rays, abdominal x-rays, C-spine series, skull series, transthoracic echo, as well as these listed below.

- Remember to restart the diet post procedure or if procedure is canceled.

Contrast Reactions

- Everyone feels a sense of warmth or flushing during contrast administration—this is not an allergy.

- For known contrast sensitivity (e.g., hives, rash), consider prednisone, 60 mg PO q6h × 4 doses prior to the exam. Diphenhydramine (Benadryl), 50 mg PO, can also be added.

- Alternatively, consider using prednisone, 60 mg PO, 12 hrs prior to procedure, then take diphenhydramine 50 mg PO + cimetidine (or other H2 receptor antagonist) 300 mg PO + prednisone 60 mg PO, when on call to the procedure.

- Although only nonionic contrast is used for CT (check your institution for confirmation), if your patient has had a major event with previous contrast administration (e.g., shock or airway compromise), discuss this with the radiologist **prior** to ordering a test. Allergic reactions generally do not occur with PO contrast.

- The contrast used in MR examinations is a gadolinium preparation, not iodinated contrast. It would be highly unusual for a patient to have an allergy to gadolinium.

Contrast Nephropathy

- This is a common complication of any procedure involving iodinated IV contrast (e.g., radiological studies, angiograms). The risk is minimal with gadolinium. Risk factors include 1) presence of chronic kidney disease, 2) diabetes, 3) larger amount of contrast infused. Strategies for prevention include:
  - IV hydration: 1 mg/kg/hr of 0.45 or 0.9 NS for 6–12 hours before and 6–12 hours after the procedure. Can also use a sodium bicarbonate solution (3 ampules of $NaHCO_3$ [150 mEq total] in 1L D5W.
  - N-acetylcysteine (Mucomyst), 600 mg bid $\times$ 2 doses before the procedure and 2 doses after the procedure, may also be added.
- Contrast should be given cautiously to anyone with a Cr >2.0.

Gastrointestinal Radiology

- GI studies can be uncomfortable and do require patient cooperation. If your patient is paralyzed, demented, angry, or has altered mental status, the study will likely be suboptimal.
- General rules for the "barium versus hypaque" dilemma (call the radiologist if you have specific questions):
  1. **Barium** is bad in pleural or peritoneal spaces so avoid this if perforation, obstruction, aspiration, or a fistula is suspected. Do not use if the patient is likely to need a laparotomy soon.
  2. **Hypaque** is bad to aspirate, so avoid in cases of possible aspiration.

TABLE 16-7.
PREPARATION FOR RADIOLOGY TESTS

PROCEDURE	PREPARATION
CT	
Chest/extremity/head	Usually none, but may need contrast
	Full liquid diet starting 4 hours prior to procedure
Abdominal/pelvic	Oral contrast administration
MRI	None
Ultrasound	
Abdominal	NPO starting 6 hours prior to procedure
Pelvic	4 glasses of water 1 hour prior; no voiding 1 hour prior

TABLE 16-7. (continued)

PROCEDURE	PREPARATION
Gastrointestinal studies	
Barium swallow (used to evaluate pharynx and esophagus typically for dysphagia work-up)	NPO 1 hour prior to procedure
Modified barium swallow (used to evaluate for possible aspiration during feeding)	NPO 1 hour prior to procedure
Upper GI (used to evaluate the esophagus, stomach, and proximal small intestine; typically used to look for ulcers)	NPO starting midnight the day of procedure
Small bowel follow-through (contrast is followed through the small intestine; typically used to evaluate for areas of stricture or large mucosal abnormalities)	1 glass of water every hour between 12 PM and 7 PM; no smoking/chewing tobacco after midnight
Barium enema (used to evaluate the colon for mucosal lesions such as polyps and strictures)	Clear liquids 1 day prior; NPO after midnight; 1 glass of water every hour from 1 PM to 7 PM 1 day prior, mag citrate at 8 PM, 4 Dulcolax tablets at 11 PM, 1 Dulcolax suppository at 7 AM
HIDA scan	NPO starting midnight the day of procedure
Genitourinary studies	
Cystogram	No dietary restriction
	Full bladder
Interventional studies	
Venogram	Clear liquids; NPO 1 hour prior to procedure
Lymphangiogram	Light meal prior; limit fluids 2–3 hours prior to procedure

TABLE 16-7. (continued)

PROCEDURE	PREPARATION
Endoscopic studies	
EGD/ERCP	NPO starting 6 hours prior to procedure
Colonoscopy	Clear liquids 1 day prior to procedure; 1 gallon of Go-LYTELY (1 cup per 15 minutes until done on night prior to procedure (consider NG tube if not able to complete); NPO after midnight
Flexible sigmoidoscopy	Clear liquids starting with dinner the night before; NPO after midnight
	Mag Citrate at 8 PM, 1 glass of water every 2 hours until 10 PM, then 3 Dulcolax tablets at 10 PM, and 1 Dulcolax suppository at 6 AM

Cardiac Studies

In general:

- No smoking 2 hours prior to test, remove nicotine patches the morning of the test.

- Small sips of water with medication are fine.

TABLE 16-8.
PREPARATION FOR CARDIAC TESTS

TEST	PREPARATION
Coronary angiogram	NPO after midnight
Stress echo, dobutamine stress echo, or exercise stress test	Take all medications (unless they need to be taken with food)
Nuclear stress test (walking)	Hold AM doses of calcium channel blockers and β-blockers

TABLE 16-8. (continued)

TEST	PREPARATION
Adenosine or dipyridamole (Persantine) nuclear stress test (non-walking)	For diabetics on insulin only, half the normal insulin dose and eat a light meal 3 hours prior to procedure (no fats or dairy products)
	Avoid any xanthine containing products (e.g., chocolate, caffeine) and theophylline or persantine for 24 hours prior to procedure

MRI

- Absolute contraindications are pacemakers and ferromagnetic intra-cranial aneurysm clips.

- Relative contraindications are recent operations (less than a few weeks) and recent vascular stenting. Prosthetic hip joints or metal implants are not generally contraindicated, but their artifact may obscure any adjacent lesions.

- As with CT, the patient must be able to lie still and cooperate—consider mild sedation (e.g., lorazepam) if necessary. Patients may get claustrophobic.

Ultrasound

- Abdominal ultrasounds can be used to evaluate the gallbladder, liver, and kidneys. The pancreas is typically not well visualized—use CT instead.

- Ultrasound can also locate pockets of fluid to guide paracentesis or thoracentesis.

- It is important the patient be made NPO as gas can obstruct the image.

17

Approach to Consultation

... With a little help from our friends ...

THE MEDICINE CONSULT

Guiding principles for effective medicine consults were first suggested by Lee Goldman and colleagues in a paper published in the *Archives of Internal Medicine* in September 1983.

The so-called 10 commandments for effective consultations are presented:

1. Determine the question being asked.

As a guiding principle, and when taking the initial phone call from the requesting service, always determine the specific medicine-related question he or she wants answered. This will be helpful, especially in situations in which the patient has an extensive and complicated previous medical history. Thus, a typical consultation note should begin by stating a specific problem, such as "Called to see this 78-year-old woman with type 2 diabetes and hypertension for perioperative glucose control..."

2. Establish urgency.

Always determine if the consult is emergent, urgent, or elective.

3. Look for yourself.

Seldom do the answers to the consultation question lie in the chart; more often than not, independent data gathering is required, including reviewing prior admissions. Often the patient requires further testing. In many cases, the data review combined with a complete history and physical exam from an internal medicine perspective will establish the diagnosis.

4. Be as brief as appropriate.

It is not necessary to repeat in detail the data already in the primary team's note; obviously as much new data independently gathered should be recorded.

5. Be specific.

Try to be goal-oriented and keep the discussion and differential diagnosis concise. When recommending drugs, always include dose, frequency, and route.

6. Provide contingency plans.

Try to anticipate potential problems (e.g., if using escalating doses of a β-blocker for rapid atrial fibrillation, make sure that regular BP checks are instituted). Staff (nursing/ancillary) on other floors are not used to treating medicine patients.

7. Honor thy turf.

Remember to answer the questions you were asked; it is not appropriate to engage the patient in a detailed discussion of whether surgery is indicated or likely to succeed. In situations in which you are asked by the patient about the surgical procedure, defer to the primary team rather than speculating on the technical aspects of the surgery.

8. Teach—with tact.

Share your insights and expertise without condescension.

9. Talk is cheap, and effective.

Communicate your recommendations directly to the requesting physician. There is no substitute for direct personal contact. Next month the shoe may be on the other foot, and the same resident may be coming to evaluate a surgical abdomen on one of your medicine admissions.

10. Follow up.

Suggestions are more likely to be translated into orders when the consultant continues to follow up.

Preoperative Cardiovascular Risk Assessment

- Preoperative evaluation and intraoperative management are aimed at eliminating or treating risk factors to reduce the risk of cardiac events (MI, unstable angina, CHF, arrhythmia, and death).

- Risk assessment guidelines have been published by the American College of Cardiology/American Heart Association Task Force (*J Am Coll Cardiol* 2002;39:542 or www.acc.org). History, physical examination, and ECG are important components of a thorough clinical assessment and help determine the extent of diagnostic testing required.

- Patients who have mild CAD on cardiac cath or successful revascularization and have no new clinical symptoms probably have a similar risk for events as patients without CAD.

- The American College of Cardiology/American Heart Association algorithm for preoperative cardiac risk assessment is detailed in Fig. 17-1.

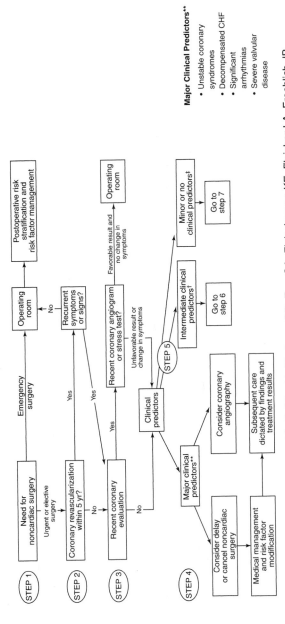

FIGURE 17-1. Eagle KA, Berger PB, Calkins H, Chaitman BR, Ewy GA, Fleischmann KE, Fleisher LA, Froehlich JB, Gusberg RJ, Leppo JA, Ryan T, Schlant RC, Wingers WL Jr. ACC/AHA guideline update for perioperative cardiovascular evaluation for noncardiac surgery: a report of the American College of Cardiology/American Heart Association Task Force on evaluation for noncardiac surgery: a report of the American College of Cardiology/American Heart Association Task Force on *(continues)*

Major Clinical Predictors**

- Unstable coronary syndromes
- Decompensated CHF
- Significant arrhythmias
- Severe valvular disease

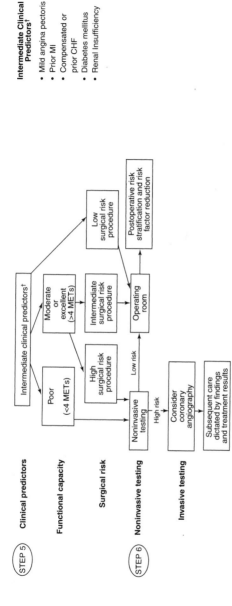

FIGURE 17-1. (*continued*) Practice Guidelines. *J Am Coll Cardiol* 2002; 39:542. METS = metabolic equivalents. 4 mets = climbing a flight of stairs or walking on level ground at 4 mph. (*continues*)

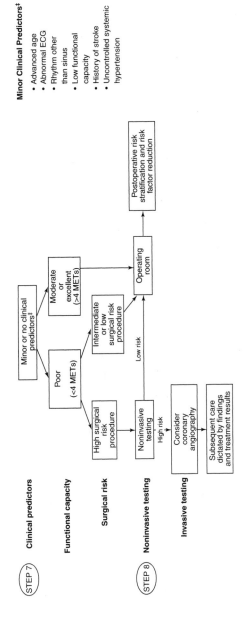

FIGURE 17-1. *(continued)*

- **β-Adrenergic antagonists** should be considered in all patients with substantial risk of cardiac disease to reduce mortality and the incidence of cardiovascular complications. Atenolol 25–100 mg PO q day or 5–10 mg IV one hour before surgery and immediately after, followed by 50–100 mg PO q day for at least 7 days afterward, are possible regimens. If the patient is already taking a β-blocker, it should be continued and titrated to a goal HR of 50–60 beats per minute.

- Angiotensin-converting enzyme inhibitors should be considered for patients with systolic heart failure.

- Patients taking calcium channel blockers should continue this medication throughout the perioperative period.

- Continuation of preoperative antihypertensive treatment throughout the perioperative period is critical, particularly if the patient is on clonidine (risk of rebound hypertension). Consider switching the patient to IV or transdermal formulations of medications if the patient will be NPO for an extended period of time.

DERMATOLOGY
Toxic Epidermal Necrolysis (TEN)

A. *Emergency—call a consult immediately!*

B. Pertinent information: drug history. Drugs are nearly always the cause. The most common offenders are sulfonamides, anticonvulsants, penicillin, NSAIDs, and allopurinol.

C. Typical symptoms: begins with fever, sore throat, burning eyes, 1–3 days before onset of skin involvement.

D. Physical exam findings: high fever, painful erythema of skin with full-thickness epidermal peeling, mucosal and conjunctival erythema.

E. Workup: CBC, blood chemistry profile, CXR, skin biopsy.

F. Diagnosis: physical exam findings and skin biopsy.

G. Treatment:

1. Stop suspect drug(s).

2. Transfer to burn unit/ICU.

3. IV Fluids, NG tube.

4. Sterile protocol, antiseptic solution, and nonadherent dressings.

5. Antibiotics only if highly suspicious of sepsis.

6. Consider IVIG.

7. Ophthalmology consult.

H. Clinical pearls: Hepatitis occurs in 10%. Most patients have anemia and lymphopenia. Neutropenia is associated with a poor prognosis. A severe drop in temperature is more indicative of sepsis than fever. Mortality approaches 30% and is most often secondary to sepsis or ARDS. Patients with HIV, systemic lupus, or a bone marrow transplant have a higher risk of developing TEN. Stevens-Johnson syndrome is also drug induced and presents with mucosal lesions and less skin involvement. Progression of painful erythema/bullae beyond 10% to 30% of the skin may indicate a transition from SJS to TEN.

Toxic Shock Syndrome

A. *Emergency—call a consult immediately!*

B. Pertinent information: age of patient, immunocompromised status, menstrual history, postsurgical.

C. Typical signs/symptoms: painful erythematous skin, sudden onset of high fever, vomiting, diarrhea, sore throat, myalgia, and hypotension.

D. Physical exam: Erythematous scarlatiniform exanthem accentuated on the trunk more than the extremities, progressing to diffuse erythema and edema, including the oral mucosa, palms, and soles. Eventually, there is desquamation of the top layer of the epidermis (not full-thickness as in TEN) in 10–12 days.

E. Workup: blood cultures, CBC, blood chemistry profile, ECG, and CXR.

F. Diagnosis: clinical (fever, typical rash, hypotension, multiorgan involvement).

G. Treatment:

   1. Remove any infected foreign bodies.

   2. IV antibiotics effective against streptococcus and penicillinase-resistant *Staphylococcus*. Clindamycin, 900 mg IV q8 hours for suspected streptococcal TSS; oxacillin 2 g IV q4 hours for suspected staphylococcal infection (or vancomycin for PCN-allergic patient). Both are usually given until culture confirms the organism.

   3. IV fluids.

   4. Consider IVIG.

   5. Monitor for hypotension/shock.

H. Clinical pearls: *Staphylococcus* scalded skin syndrome has a similar clinical picture; however, it occurs in immunocompromised adults. *S. aureus* is the most common cause of TSS; however, exotoxin-producing streptococci can induce a similar clinical picture associated with higher mortality. Clindamycin suppresses synthesis of the TSS toxin (TSST-1) while beta-lacatamase resistant antibiotics may increase synthesis of TSST-1. Therefore, the addition of clindamycin (for the first few days of therapy) is recommended with staphylococcal infections.

Necrotizing Fasciitis

A. *Emergency—call a surgeon now!*

B. Pertinent info: recent surgical or traumatic wound.

C. Typical signs and symptoms: Involved area becomes erythematous, indurated, and severely painful. Within hours it can become dusky blue to black, indicating necrosis. Crepitus can develop because of subcutaneous gas formation.

D. Workup and diagnosis: culture and sensitivity of wound aspirate, plain x-ray for soft tissue gas, and CT/MRI if clinical diagnosis not obvious or to delineate depth of infection.

E. Treatment:

   1. Wide surgical debridement.

   2. IV antibiotics effective against gram-negative bacilli, streptococci, and anaerobes. Consider agents effective against MRSA, if in an endemic area.

F. Clinical pearls: Time is essential—*call for help immediately!*

Pemphigus Vulgaris (PV) and Bullous Pemphigoid (BP)

A. Urgent consult.

B. Pertinent info: flaccid or tense bullae, percentage body involved, mucosal involvement.

C. Typical signs and symptoms: flaccid bullae with mucosal involvement (PV) and pruritus with tense bullae in an elderly person (BP).

D. Workup and diagnosis: skin biopsy with direct immunofluorescence and serum for indirect immunofluorescence.

E. Treatment:

   1. PV: prednisone, azathioprine, mycophenolate mofetil, gold.

   2. BP: steroids (topical > systemic), tetracycline, nicotinamide.

F. Clinical pearls: PV is associated with a higher mortality than BP. Thus, PV requires aggressive treatment. Most patients do not require hospitalization unless infected or having difficulty maintaining fluid intake. Causes of blistering diseases include infectious, autoimmune, allergic hypersensitivity, metabolic, and genetic.

Vasculitis

A. Urgent consult.

B. Pertinent info: drug history, known connective tissue disease, malignancy, or infection.

C. Typical skin findings: palpable purpura (dark reddish-brown lesions that do not blanch and may blister or ulcerate) on the lower extremities or dependent areas.

D. Workup: CBC, blood chemistry profile, urinalysis, Hemoccult, skin biopsy, CXR, throat culture for strep, ESR, hepatitis panel, cryoglobulins, ANA, RF, antiphospholipid, ANCA, SPEP.

E. Diagnosis: skin biopsy; concern for systemic involvement if fever, arthralgias, abdominal pain, pulmonary symptoms, hematuria, or proteinuria.

F. Treatment:

1. Discontinue potential causative drug (ASA, sulfonamides, penicillin, barbiturates, amphetamines, PTU).

2. Treat underlying disorder (infection, malignancy, or connective tissue disease).

3. Antihistamines, NSAIDs, colchicine, dapsone, antimalarials.

4. If systemic involvement: prednisone, azathioprine, cyclophosphamide, IVIG, plasmapheresis.

G. Clinical pearls: 50% of cases are idiopathic. Thrombocytopenia is associated with nonpalpable purpura. DIC and coumadin necrosis cause extensive purpura. *Neisseria* sepsis and Rocky Mountain spotted fever also cause petechiae and purpura. Acral hemorrhagic papules, pustules, or vesicles may result from septic emboli.

Hypersensitivity Syndrome (Severe Drug Reaction)

A. Urgent consult.

B. Pertinent information: drug history (sulfonamides, anticonvulsants, allopurinol).

C. Physical exam: maculopapular blanching eruption, exfoliative dermatitis, or erythema multiforme-like lesions mostly on the trunk and proximal extremities, fever, lymphadenopathy, hepatosplenomegaly.

D. Workup: CBC, liver function panel, urinalysis, CXR.

E. Treatment:

1. Stop drug.

2. Oral steroids and antihistamines for symptoms.

F. Clinical pearls: The syndrome develops within 8 weeks of starting the causative drug. Up to 50% develop fulminant hepatic necrosis if the drug is not stopped early in the course. Some anticonvulsants cross-react in 70% to 80% of patients (phenytoin, carbamazepine, and phenobarbital). Patients should warn first-degree relatives that they, too, may be at high risk for a reaction to these anticonvulsants.

Erythroderma

A. Urgent consult.

B. Pertinent info: prior skin disorder, drug history, duration of erythroderma.

C. Physical exam: diffuse erythema of skin leading to exfoliative dermatitis, pruritus, keratoderma, shivering/chills, alopecia.

D. Labs: CBC, blood chemistry panel, albumin, calcium, SPEP, peripheral blood smear for Sézary cells.

E. Diagnosis: clinical, skin biopsy.

F. Treatment:

1. Treat underlying skin condition if known (psoriasis, eczema, etc.).

2. Discontinue suspect drugs if any.

3. Search for and treat underlying malignancy.

4. Topical steroid ointment (midpotency), emollients, systemic antihistamines.

5. Monitor closely for electrolyte and fluid imbalances, high-output cardiac failure, renal failure, sepsis, and hypothermia.

G. Clinical pearls: 20% of cases are idiopathic. The course and prognosis depend on the underlying etiology. A diligent search for the underlying cause is often required. Most patients do not require hospitalization unless infected or in high-output cardiac failure.

NEUROLOGY
Stroke

A. If stroke is suspected, the level of urgency is guided by the time of onset. *If the neurologic deficit occurred within three hours and is persisting or worsening, call a consultation immediately.* TIAs (ischemic deficits that clear in less than 24 hours, usually within 5–10 minutes require urgent consultation and attention.

B. General points:

1. When to suspect this:

   a. An acute neurologic deficit that falls within a cerebral vascular territory.

   b. A neurologic deficit involving the loss of speech, cognition, movement, sensation, or vision.

2. What isn't a stroke:

   a. Noncirculatory neurologic problems that appear suddenly or may be noticed relatively acutely that on further questioning reveal themselves to be subacute or chronic.

   b. Positive neurologic symptoms such as pain are unusual.

   c. Syncope, seizure with postictal (Todd's) paralysis, isolated dizziness, memory loss, and confusion (rule out aphasia) have all been mistaken for strokes.

3. Classification:

   a. Hemorrhage (nontraumatic, intraparenchymal, or subarachnoid).

   b. Ischemic stroke.

C. Pertinent information:

1. Time course of symptoms (gradual or sudden?).

2. Exact time of onset. When was the patient last known to be normal?

3. Progression of symptoms: Improving, worsening, or staying the same?

4. Did the patient fall?

5. Associated symptoms? Headache, neck pain, nausea, and vomiting suggest hemorrhagic stroke.

6. Are there contraindications for giving acute thrombolytic therapy? Contraindications include: (a) >3 hours since onset of symptoms; (b) extensive infarct on CT scan; (c) recent surgery or head trauma; (d) recent MI; (e) recent GI or urinary hemorrhage; (f) bleeding diatheses or anticoagulation; (g) uncontrolled hypertension (SBP >185, DBP >110); (h) seizure at stroke onset.

7. Neurologic, general medical, and recent surgical history.

8. Patient's medications including anticoagulation.

D. Physical exam:

1. Vital signs: Blood pressure, pulse, respirations, and temperature; finger-stick glucose level, oxygen saturation.

2. Signs of head injury.

3. Observe for oral trauma that would suggest an unwitnessed seizure.

4. Cardiopulmonary exam focusing on possible arrhythmia, congestive heart failure, aspiration.

5. Focused neurologic exam.

E. Workup:

1. Stat noncontrast CT of the head to differentiate between a hemorrhagic and an ischemic stroke.

2. Basic studies should be obtained such as an ECG, CXR, finger-stick glucose, CBC, chemistry panel, PT, PTT, and urinalysis.

F. Treatment:

1. Intracerebral hemorrhage

a. Initial management is directed toward the basic ABCs.

i. Protect the airway and provide oxygenation.

ii. Intubation should be considered for anyone with:

- Decreasing level of consciousness.

- Signs of brain stem dysfunction.

- Insufficient ventilation as indicated by hypoxia (Po_2 <60 mm Hg or Pco_2 >50 mm Hg) or obvious risk for aspiration regardless of arterial oxygenation.

b. Blood pressure management.

i. Hypertension.

- Avoid overaggressive treatment of elevated blood pressure.

- Consider antihypertensive therapy only if mean arterial BP >130 (or systolic BP is >220 mm Hg and diastolic BP >120 mm Hg) or evidence of other end-organ involvement (e.g., MI, pulmonary edema, aortic dissection).

- Commonly used antihypertensive medications are labetalol, 10–40 mg IV boluses q hour and hydralazine, 10–20 mg IV q4–6h.

    ii. Treat hypotension (systolic arterial blood pressure <90 mm Hg or below relative baseline).

- Volume replenishment with isotonic saline is first line.

- If hypotension persists after correction of volume deficit, pressors should be considered, especially if systolic pressure is <90 mm Hg.

- Commonly used pressors are phenylephrine, 2–10 μg/kg/min, dopamine, 2–20 μg/kg/min, and norepinephrine, 0.05–0.2 μg/kg/min.

2. Ischemic stroke

    a. **Thrombolytic Treatment: Time is Brain**! The only FDA-approved treatment for acute ischemic stroke is thrombolytic therapy, which must be given within 3 hours from time of onset before the risk of symptomatic hemorrhage exceeds the benefit of thrombolysis. *Obtain an immediate consultation if you think the patient may qualify for treatment with thrombolytic therapy.*

    b. Blood pressure management.

       i. In practice, treatment is less aggressive in ischemic stroke.

       ii. Consider only if systolic BP is >220 mm Hg or diastolic BP >120 mm Hg, or if thrombolytic medication is considered or in the presence of other hypertensive crises.

       iii. Treat hypotension.

Seizures

A. Level of urgency/emergency:

- *Status epilepticus is an emergency. Call a consult immediately*!

- New onset of a single seizure requires an immediate assessment into its causes.

- A single seizure recurrence in a patient with a known seizure disorder may need an urgent consult depending on its course and severity.

B. Factors that may influence a more **urgent** consultation:

- Failure to regain cognition and function after the seizure.

- Seizure type or severity atypical for the patient.

C. Important historical information:

- Has mental status returned?

- Describe the seizure. Are the movements rhythmic, asynchronous, one side involved more than the other, head turning left or right?

- Known seizure disorder?

- Known metabolic disorder?

D. Physical exam: signs of head injury, oropharyngeal trauma, signs of meningismus, arrhythmia, occurrence of aspiration, neurologic exam with focus on the level of consciousness, any focal signs of cranial nerve impairment and motor or sensory loss.

E. Workup information:

1. A seizure is a symptom; search for an etiology (consider structural causes, infections, stroke, trauma, metabolic, iatrogenic, neoplastic).

2. Labs include fingerstick glucose, Na, Ca, Mg, Phos, and BUN/Cr.

F. Treatment:

1. What to do when a patient is having a seizure:

   a. Remain calm. Determine if the patient is still having a seizure.

   b. Take measures to protect the patient.

      i. Place the patient in the lateral decubitus position with suctioning nearby.

      ii. Pad the bed rails to avoid head injury.

      iii. Remove sharp and hard objects that may potentially cause injury.

   c. Attend to the ABCs.

      i. Provide oxygen by cannula or nonrebreather face mask.

      ii. Protect the airway.

      iii. Obtain vital signs.

      iv. Obtain a fingerstick glucose.

2. If the patient is still having seizures, either continuous activity lasting >5 minutes or two or more discrete seizures between which there is incomplete recovery of consciousness, status epilepticus has developed. Note that two seizures between which there is recovery of consciousness does not define status.

Status Epilepticus

A. *Emergency—call a consult immediately!*

B. Definition: Continuous seizure for >5 minutes or two or more discrete seizures with incomplete recovery of consciousness.

C. Treatment:

1. Ensure adequate respiration (100% O_2 by mask); have airway box/suction at bedside available; have intubation kit ready.

2. Establish ECG monitor, continuous pulse oximetry, and ABG.

3. NG tube placement.

4. Obtain vitals including temperature.

5. Ensure IV access.

6. Labs: Obtain fingerstick glucose, serum chemistries including Na, Ca, Mg, phos, serum and urine toxicology screens, EtOH level, UA, drug levels, and CBC.

7. Give 50 mL of 50% glucose and thiamine, 100 mg IVP. Untreated hypoglycemia has much more serious consequences than transient hyperglycemia.

8. Administer lorazepam (Ativan), 0.1 mg/kg IV (4–8 mg at a maximum of 2 mg/min); if no IV access, rectal diazepam, 0.5 mg/kg.

9. Phenytoin IV, 15–20 mg/kg (in dextrose-free solution) at a rate of 1 mg/kg/min to a maximum of 50 mg/min (monitor BP and cardiac rhythm). Alternatively, fosphenytoin IV, 15–20 mg phenytoin equivalents/kg, can be used. It tends to be safer with less risk of hypotension.

10. **Persistent refractory status:** If seizures continue >60 minutes.

    a. Intubation and transfer to an ICU with continuous EEG monitoring.

    b. Pentobarbital, 5–12 mg/kg bolus then infusion 1.5 mg/kg/hr increased q5–10min until status stopped or flat EEG obtained.

    c. Midazolam, 0.2 mg/kg IV bolus then 0.1–0.6 mg/kg/hr: Induces less hypotension and cardiorespiratory depression and can be easily titrated; however, tachyphylaxis is a problem.

    d. Propofol, 3–5 mg/kg bolus, then infusion at 1–15 mg/kg/hr.

11. When IV access is not available:

    a. Rectal diazepam at 0.5 mg/kg (maximum 20 mg).

    b. Intramuscular midazolam, 0.2 mg/kg bolus (mean time to peak serum concentration 25 minutes).

    c. Intranasal midazolam; usually terminates within 10 minutes of administration (0.15–0.3 mg/kg).

D. Clinical pearls:

1. Treat the underlying cause and optimize dose of medications.

2. Urine dipstick to detect myoglobin to watch for rhabdomyolysis.

3. Treat hyperthermia (40°C core) with a cooling blanket, antipyretics.

Bacterial Meningitis

A. Level of urgency/emergency. When suspected, urgent evaluation is required for prompt diagnosis and treatment, and can minimize the neurologic complications following acute bacterial meningitis.

B. When to suspect this:

- History of myalgias, ear pain, sore throat, joint stiffness, fatigue occurring several days before major clinical deterioration is often noted.

- Fever and vomiting are the most consistent early signs, present in more than three-fourths of patients.

- Headache, often described as bursting and splitting, is severe enough to overcome the most commonly prescribed medications. Photophobia may be present.

- Altered level of consciousness occurs in most patients, varying from delirium to drowsiness and stupor. An acute confusional state in a febrile elderly patient, for example, should always raise the possibility of acute bacterial meningitis and should not be assumed to have resulted from a pneumonia or urinary tract infection.

- In HIV and other immunocompromised patients, fungal infections such as cryptococcus also should be considered.

C. Physical exam:

1. Seizures may develop at some point in the course of the disease.

2. Careful neurologic exam is essential. Flexion of the neck that results in spontaneous flexion of the knees (Brudzinski's sign) and passive extension of the knees while the hips are flexed results in eye opening and a verbal response (Kernig's sign).

3. Papilledema may suggest superior sagittal sinus thrombosis or progressive brain edema.

4. Rash (petechial or purpuric) suggests *Neisseria meningitidis*, less often *Staphylococcus aureus*, pneumococcus, or rickettsiae.

D. Workup:

1. Blood cultures and urgent lumbar puncture are required. See Table 17-1 for CSF analysis.

2. Obtain a head CT before LP to rule out a mass effect as a cause of the altered level of consciousness, especially if there is a finding of focality or increased intracranial pressure.

3. When CT cannot be done in a timely fashion, blood cultures should be obtained and empiric antibiotic therapy started. See Table 17-2 for treatment options. CT should then be performed followed by urgent LP afterward.

Viral Meningitis

A. This is an urgent consultation. Prognosis depends on rapid diagnosis and stage of the illness when treatment is begun.

B. Symptoms: altered consciousness, fever, change in personality, headache, a flu-like illness may precede initial symptoms by a few days.

C. Physical exam: assess mental status, focusing on level of consciousness, language, and memory. Look for signs of autonomic dysfunction.

D. Diagnosis:

1. If HSV is suspected, start acyclovir (see Treatment section) while diagnostic studies are pending.

2. MRI: More sensitive than CT and is therefore the first choice. T2 hyperintensity of the temporal and orbitofrontal lobes may be present.

3. CT may be normal early or show signs of low attenuation in the anterior and mesial temporal lobes.

4. CSF studies: Do not do LP if evidence of mass effect.

   • CSF is normal in 5% to 10% of cases. Refer to Table 17-1 for more information.

   • CSF PCR: Highly sensitive (95%) and specific; remains positive up to 5 days after starting acyclovir.

5. EEG: Usually abnormal.

E. Treatment:

1. Acyclovir 10 mg/kg IV q8h × 10–14 days if diagnosis of HSV is confirmed. Monitor and follow renal function closely in patients with renal impairment.

TABLE 17-1.
CSF ANALYSIS

Condition	Color	Pressure (mm H$_2$O)	Cells (No./mL)	Protein (mg/dL)	Glucose (mg/dL)
Normal	Clear	70–180	0–5 mononuclear	15–45	45–80 (two-thirds of serum glucose)
Bacterial meningitis	Opalescent	Increased (may be normal)	>5 to many 1,000 PMNs	50–1,500	0–45
Viral infection	Clear or opalescent	Normal (may be slightly increased)	>5–2,000, mostly lymphs	20–200	Normal (may be slightly decreased)
Tuberculous meningitis	Clear or opalescent	Increased (may be normal)	>5–500 lymphs	45–500	10–45
Fungal meningitis	Clear or opalescent	Normal or increased	>5–800 lymphs	Normal or increased	Normal or decreased
Carcinomatous meningitis	Clear or opalescent	Normal or increased	>5–1,000 mononuclear	Up to 500	Normal or decreased
Subarachnoid hemorrhage	Bloody or xanthochromic	Increased (may be normal)	Many RBC; ratio of WBC/RBC same as blood	Up to 2,000	Normal

TABLE 17-2.
TREATMENT OPTIONS FOR BACTERIAL MENINGITIS

Age or clinical setting	Likely organism	Empiric treatment
Immunocompetent		
18–50 years	*Streptococcus pneumoniae, Neisseria meningitidis*	Third generation cephalosporin
>50 years	*S. pneumoniae, L. monocytogenes*, gram-negative bacilli	Third generation cephalosporin + ampicillin
TB	*Mycobacterium tuberculosis*	Isoniazid + rifampin + ethambutol + pyrazinamide
Head trauma, CSF shunt, neurosurgery	Staphylococci, gram-negative bacilli, *S. pneumoniae*	Vancomycin + ceftazidime
Immunocompromised	*L. monocytogenes*, gram-negative bacilli, also *S. pneumoniae* and *Haemophilus influenzae*	Ampicillin + ceftazidime
HIV	*Cryptococcus neoforms*	Amphotericin B + flucytosine

2. If a temporal lobe lesion typical of HSV is present along with edema on head imaging, reduce ICP (20 mg bolus of dexamethasone IV, then 4 mg q4h). If mass effect produces a midline shift >3 mm or the patient deteriorates or is comatose, intubate, and hyperventilate to a P_{CO_2} of 28–30 mm Hg. If herniation is impending, IV mannitol, 50–100 g, should be given.

F. Clinical pearls:

1. Prompt recognition and treatment of suspected cases minimizes neurologic complications.

2. HSV encephalitis makes up approximately 10% to 20% of adult cases of acute encephalitis.

3. Positive predictors of bacterial meningitis (99% PPV):

- Glucose <34 mg/dL

- Protein >200 mg/dL

- CSF/serum glucose <0.23

- WBC $>2,000/mm^3$
- PMNs $>1,180/mm^3$

Neuroleptic Malignant Syndrome

A. Urgent consult.

B. When to suspect:

1. May arise during early treatment with neuroleptic therapy, most often when doses are increased quickly or from a previously well-tolerated neuroleptic.

2. Dehydration and hyponatremia may be predisposing factors.

3. Has the patient been on other medications such as selective serotonin reuptake inhibitors, tetrabenazine, or acutely withdrawn from an antiparkinsonian medication?

C. History and physical exam: Fever, extreme rigidity, dysautonomia, depressed level of consciousness, tremor, dystonia, and other dyskinesias are prominent.

D. Workup:

1. Diagnosis is primarily by history.

2. An elevated CK level is nonspecific but may help with the diagnosis.

3. Other considerations include meningitis, encephalitis, systemic infection, heat stroke, and malignant hyperthermia.

E. Treatment:

1. Withdraw the neuroleptic immediately.

2. Mortality results from complications of hyperthermia.

3. Treat hyperthermia aggressively with antipyretics and cooling blanket.

4. Consider dantrolene (1–2 mg/kg IV up to 10 mg/kg maximum), followed by 4–8 mg/kg in four divided doses per day for 3 days.

5. Monitor frequently for autonomic dysfunction.

6. Manage fluid status and electrolytes.

OBSTETRICS AND GYNECOLOGY
Key Points

A. Obtain a menstrual history including LMP, pregnancy status, age at menarche, duration between menses, length of menses, amount of vaginal bleeding (i.e., how many pads soaked in how many hours?).

B. Also ask about last Pap smear, history of abnormal Pap smear results, history of any postmenopausal bleeding.

C. Obtain an obstetric history: Gravida and para status (including full-term deliveries, premature deliveries, stillbirths, abortions or miscarriages, and living children).

D. Obtain a sexual history including form of contraception, number of partners, bleeding with intercourse, and history of sexually transmitted diseases.

E. Perform a physical exam including a pelvic exam. If access to a speculum or pelvic table is limited, then a bimanual and rectovaginal exam can be performed at the bedside.

Ectopic Pregnancy

A. *Emergency—call a consult immediately!*

B. History: Date of patient's LMP, menstrual history, type of contraception (if any), history of tubal ligation, history of ectopic pregnancy, amount of vaginal bleeding (if any), and degree of abdominal pain (if any). *Note: History of a tubal ligation does not by any means rule out an ectopic pregnancy.*

C. Physical exam: Take **vital signs immediately** with orthostatics and fetal heart tones auscultated by Doppler.

D. Workup: Tests to be drawn include CBC, type and screen, and urine pregnancy test (if positive, draw a quantitative β-hCG immediately).

E. Treatment:

1. Place large-bore IV immediately.

2. The gynecologic consult team should be notified **immediately** if:

   • Pregnancy test result is positive

   • No fetal heart tones are heard

   • History of vaginal bleeding or abdominal pain

3. If there is a positive pregnancy test result and hemodynamic instability exists, resuscitation with blood and prompt surgical exploration is necessary.

Vaginal Bleeding

A. *Heavy vaginal bleeding can be an emergency—call a consult immediately!* Type and cross the patient if the bleeding is heavy, the patient is unstable, or both, and make sure a pregnancy test has been done and large-bore IV has been placed.

B. History:

- Assess how long the bleeding has lasted, where the patient is in her cycle, how much bleeding has occurred, if there is a history of bleeding disorders, and whether the patient is on hormones, contraception, or anticoagulants, and when she last took any of these medications or if any of the medication has been recently changed. Determine by history whether the bleeding is chronic or acute.

- Assess risk factors for cervical cancer (history of abnormal Pap smear results, smoking, multiparity, low socioeconomic group, number of sexual partners, age at first intercourse, history of cervical cancer).

- Assess risk factors for endometrial cancer (obesity, diabetes, hypertension, unopposed estrogen consumption, history of abnormal endometrial biopsies, early age at menarche or late age at menopause, history of anovulation, family history of endometrial cancer or history of colon or breast cancer).

C. Physical exam: Determine source of bleeding—make sure the bleeding is from the vagina or uterus and not the urethra (inspect the urethra), bladder (do a straight catheterization), or rectum (rectal exam).

D. Workup: Pregnancy test (if positive, do a type and screen for Rh status and the need for RhoGAM for **all** patients), CBC.

E. Treatment:

1. Place large-bore IV.

2. Rehydration with fluids; transfuse with pRBC if unstable.

3. D/C any anticoagulants.

4. Notify Ob/Gyn consultant.

Pelvic Mass

A. *Call a gynecology consult immediately for suspected ovarian torsion.* Other causes do not require emergent consultation.

B. History: Obtain a thorough history including menstrual history, menopausal status, pregnancy status, history of neoplasia, history of vaginal bleeding, last Pap smear, history or recent biopsy of any gynecologic organs, and history of any gynecologic surgery. Ask about family history of ovarian, breast, or colon cancer, and history of tobacco use.

C. Physical exam: Perform pelvic exam (including speculum exam) to thoroughly visualize the cervix, bimanual and rectovaginal exam to assess motility, position, and further characterize the mass.

D. Workup: Radiologic exams include abdominal/pelvic CT (determine the position in relation to other pelvic organs [adnexa, uterus, cervix], size of the mass, if the mass is complex, fluid- or blood-filled areas, and whether calcifications are present). Patient may need a pelvic ultrasound.

E. Clinical pearls: The differential diagnosis includes neoplasms and benign cysts but may also involve ovarian torsion. Torsion may present as a pelvic mass but is usually accompanied by intermittent severe abdominal pain, tender pelvic mass by exam, low-grade temperatures, and on pelvic ultrasound may be accompanied by decreased flow to the ovary.

OPHTHALMOLOGY
Trauma with Possible Ruptured Globe

A. *Ocular emergency—call a consult immediately!*

B. Pertinent information: age, PMH/PSH/ocular history, allergies, current meds including ocular meds, specific ocular complaints, history of events preceding trauma, specific chemicals or items involved.

C. Typical symptoms: pain, decreased vision, history of trauma.

D. Physical exam findings: 360-degree subconjunctival heme, full thickness corneal or scleral laceration, irregular pupil, exposed intraocular contents, hyphema.

E. Treatment:

1. Place a shield over the involved eye; **do not touch ocular contents**.

2. NPO (determine last meal).

3. IV antibiotics: cefazolin or ceftazidime or vancomycin 1 gm IV immediately.

4. Orbital CT scan (axial and coronal).

5. Surgical repair within 24 hours.

F. Clinical pearls:

1. In trauma with eyelid laceration; do NOT try to repair the laceration. Allow ophthalmologist to assess extent.

2. If there is severe eyelid swelling, this is a possible sign of orbital cellulitis.

3. Significant orbital trauma may require evaluation for retrobulbar heme, optic nerve trauma, and fractures.

Injury

Acute Chemical Splash

A. *Ocular emergency*—begin irrigation, *then call a consult immediately.*

B. Pertinent information: age, PMH/PSH/ocular history, allergies, current meds including ocular meds, specific ocular complaints, history of events, specific chemicals or items involved, time, irrigation.

C. Symptoms: ± pain, blurry vision, foreign body sensation, tearing, photophobia.

D. Physical exam:

1. Mild to moderate splash: Sloughing of entire epithelium, hyperemia, mild chemosis, eyelid edema, first or second degree periocular skin burns.

2. Moderate to severe: Pronounced chemosis, perilimbal blanching, corneal edema or opacification, anterior chamber reaction/no view of the anterior chamber, increased intraocular pressure, second or third degree burns.

E. Workup: Slit-lamp exam, evert eyelids, check pH, intraocular pressure.

F. Immediate treatment:

1. *Copious irrigation* with 1 L of any available irrigant (e.g., NS, ½ NS, or LR), and keep irrigating until you talk with the consultant.

2. May give 1–2 drops of topical anesthetic.

3. Do *not* use acid or alkali to neutralize splash.

4. Check pH 5 minutes after irrigation.

G. Treatment *after* irrigation:

1. Debride necrotic tissue

2. Topical antibiotic ointment: bacitracin/polymyxin (Polysporin), erythromycin, or ciprofloxacin (Ciloxan) ophthalmic qid

3. Cycloplege the eye with homatropine 5% bid (avoid phenylephrine)

4. Topical steroid: prednisolone 1% (Pred Forte or Pred Mild) qid

5. Pressure patch

6. Antiglaucoma drops: timolol (Timoptic) 0.5% or brimonidine (Alphagan) 0.2% bid prn

7. Daily follow-up with ophthalmology, gradual taper of steroids

Corneal Ulcer

A. *This is an emergency—call a consult immediately.*

B. Pertinent information: age, past ocular history, history leading up to event (recent trauma or contact lens use).

C. Symptoms: pain, photophobia, decreased vision, $\pm$ discharge.

D. Physical exam: focal opacity/overlying epithelial defect, anterior chamber reaction, hypopyon (pus behind eye), eyelid edema.

E. Workup: Gram's stain and fungal culture, *E. coli* overlay.

F. Treatment:

1. Ofloxacin (Ocuflox) drops, q2–4h, and cycloplege with homatropine 5% bid.

2. If ulcer is severe: admit and give fortified cefazolin (Ancef), 50 mg/mL, q hour and tobramycin, 15 mg/mL drops q hour.

G. Clinical pearls: Contact lens wearers are at much higher risk. Bacteria, fungi, HSV, and *Acanthamoeba* are all possible causes.

Corneal Abrasion or Foreign Body

A. This is usually not an emergency, but consult if in doubt.

B. Pertinent information: age, past ocular history, history of events leading up to event, occupational history (i.e., grinding, drilling, trauma), contact lens use, type of foreign body.

C. Symptoms: acute pain, tearing, photophobia.

D. Workup:

1. Blue light or slit-lamp exam with fluorescein to detect epithelial irregularities.

2. Look for foreign body or rust ring.

3. Measure and record dimension of irregularities.

4. Evert eyelids to look for hidden foreign bodies.

5. Look for associated corneal ulcers.

E. Treatment:

1. Remove foreign body (preferably by an ophthalmologist).

2. Noncontact lens wearers: Cycloplege with homatropine 5% bid, treat with bacitracin/polymyxin (Polysporin), or erythromycin ointment tid, patch eye.

3. Contact lens wearers: *no* patch, treat with ciprofloxacin opthalmic (Ciloxan) 0.3% qid × 7 days.

4. Follow up next day with an ophthalmologist and close follow-up as needed thereafter.

F. Clinical pearls: If you remove corneal metallic foreign bodies, make sure there is no rust ring left behind. If there is any chance of penetrating injury, call a consult immediately.

Acute Vision Loss
Central Retinal Artery Occlusion

A. *Ocular emergency—call a consult STAT!*

B. Pertinent information: age, PMH/PSH/ocular history, allergies, current meds including ocular meds, specific ocular complaints, history preceding event, vision loss.

C. Symptoms: painless, unilateral, acute loss of vision, prior history of amaurosis fugax.

D. Physical exam: whitening of the retina with a "cherry red" spot in the center of the macula, afferent pupillary defect (Marcus Gunn pupil), narrowed arterioles, occasionally arteriolar emboli/plaque visible.

E. Workup: ESR, fasting blood sugar, CBC, PT/PTT, ANA, RF, RPR/FTA- Ab. Check blood pressure, carotid dopplers, cardiac echo.

F. Treatment:

1. Call opthalmologist!

2. Ocular massage (direct digital massage or with fundus contact lens). Apply pressure for 5–15 seconds, then release. Repeat several times.

3. Antiglaucoma drops such as timolol (Timoptic), apraclonidine (Iopidine), dorzolamide (Trusopt), latanoprost (Xalatan), and/or acetazolamide (Diamox), 500 mg PO × 1.

G. Clinical pearls: Etiology can be embolic (carotid or cardiac), thrombosis, giant cell arteritis, collagen vascular disease, hypercoagulable disorders (i.e., SLE, PAN), retinal detachment, or rare causes (i.e., migraines, Behçet's syndrome, syphilis).

Acute Angle-Closure Glaucoma

A. *Ocular emergency—call consult immediately!*

B. Pertinent information: age, PMH/PSH/ocular history, allergies, current meds including ocular meds, specific ocular complaints, family history, recent surgery, recent laser surgery.

C. Symptoms: Pain, blurry vision, colored halos around lights, frontal headache, nausea/vomiting.

D. Physical exam: Beefy red conjunctival injection, fixed, mid-dilated pupil (usually in one eye), shallow anterior chamber, acutely elevated intraocular pressure (40s or above!).

E. Workup: Slit-lamp exam, measure intraocular pressure.

F. Treatment:

1. Topical anti-glaucoma drops (timolol [Timoptic], brimonidine [Alphagan], dorzolamide [Trusopt], latanoprost [Xalatan]).

2. Topical steroid prednisolone (Pred Forte) 1% q15min × 4 doses.

3. Carbonic anhydrase inhibitor IV or PO (i.e., acetazolamide [Diamox] 250 mg IV).

4. Osmotic agent (isosorbide, mannitol, glycerin).

5. If patient is phakic, give pilocarpine 1%–2%; if aphakic, use cycloplegic agent such as cyclopentolate 1%–2%.

6. Definitive (laser) treatment by ophthalmologist.

G. Clinical pearls: Be aware of patient's cardiovascular and pulmonary status, evaluate electrolyte/renal status before starting carbonic anhydrase inhibitors or osmotic agents. Etiology can be from an anatomic pupillary block, neovascular, anterior displacement of lens-iris diaphragm (i.e., choroidals, tumor), malignant glaucoma, medications (i.e., mydriatics, anticholinergics).

Papilledema (*Disc Edema Secondary to Increased Intracranial Pressure*)

A. *Ocular emergency—call a consult immediately!*

B. Pertinent information: age, PMH/PSH/ocular history, allergies, current meds including ocular meds, specific ocular complaints, history of events preceding trauma.

C. Symptoms: transient vision loss, headache, nausea/vomiting, diplopia, scotomata.

D. Physical exam: bilateral swollen, hyperemic discs, blurring of disc margins, obscured vessels, cotton-wool spots, dilated/tortuous veins, normal pupillary response, and color vision.

E. Workup: Check BP, careful ocular exam (pupils, color vision, exam of fundus), urgent orbital and head CT. Consider LP (after head CT), CBC, TSH, ESR. Consider a neurology consult.

F. Treatment:

1. Treat underlying cause!

G. Clinical pearls: Etiologies you may see on a medical service include pseudotumor cerebri, subdural/subarachnoid hemorrhage, AVM or sagittal sinus thrombosis, intracranial tumors, brain abscess, meningitis/encephalitis, hydrocephalus, malignant HTN, uveitis, infiltrative disease (i.e., sarcoid, TB, syphilis), ischemic optic neuropathy (i.e., giant cell arteritis), central retinal vein occlusion, papillitis (i.e., multiple sclerosis/optic neuritis, diabetic eye disease). It is often helpful to communicate the level of confidence of your fundus exam to the consultant.

Retinal Detachment

A. *Ocular urgency—call a consult.*

B. Pertinent information: age, PMH/PSH/ocular history, allergies, current meds, specific complaints, history of preceding trauma or surgery.

C. Symptoms: Painless unilateral decreased vision with associated flashes and floaters, curtain or veil across vision, relative visual field defect.

D. Physical exam: typically a "white & quiet"—appearing eye—externally looks normal, usually *no* afferent pupillary defect unless a large retinal detachment. Fundus exam reveals a white, billowing, or wrinkled retina.

E. Workup: Slit-lamp exam and dilated fundus exam.

F. Treatment:

1. No acute intervention.

2. Low level activity.

3. Needs a retina specialist evaluation.

G. Clinical pearls: Risk factors include recent eye surgery, ocular trauma, high myopia, and a retinal detachment in contralateral eye. A peripheral retinal tear or hole may present with only flashes or floaters and no change in vision. These still require urgent ophthalmologic intervention.

Infection

Endophthalmitis (Infection of the Inside of the Eye)

A. *Ocular emergency—call a consult immediately!*

B. Pertinent information: age, PMH/PSH/ocular history, allergies, current meds including ocular meds, history of ocular surgery or trauma.

C. Symptoms: unilateral painful eye, decreased vision.

D. Physical exam: moderate injection, hypopyon (pus behind the cornea), poor red reflex or view to the back of the eye.

E. Treatment:

1. Emergent ophthalmologic evaluation.

2. Admission.

3. IV vancomycin 1 gm q12h + ceftazidime 1 gm q12h.

4. May need culture and injected antibiotics.

F. Clinical pearls: A diagnosis of endophthalmitis must be considered *first* in any patient with recent ocular surgery!

Herpes Simplex

A. This is not an ocular emergency, but urgent referral to ophthalmologist is strongly recommended.

B. Pertinent information: age, PMH, ocular history, possible mode of transmission.

C. Symptoms: usually unilateral, pain, tearing, photophobia.

D. Physical exam: skin vesicles, conjunctival injection and follicles, dendritic keratitis, iritis, uveitis, retinitis.

E. Treatment:

1. Trifluridine ophthalmic (Viroptic) 1% or Vira A ointment 5 times per day for 7 days.

2. Acyclovir, 200 mg PO 5 times per day or valacyclovir (Valtrex), 500 mg PO tid.

3. Homatropine 5% drops bid.

4. Prednisolone (Pred Forte) 1% drops qid (do NOT give steroids with epithelial disease).

5. Empiric coverage with bacitracin/polymyxin (Polysporin) drops qid is recommended.

6. Follow up next day with ophthalmologist.

F. Clinical pearls: If herpetic lesions are found in distribution of cranial nerve V_1, follow closely for involvement of the eye.

The Red Eye

Conjunctivitis

A. This is not an emergency.

B. Pertinent information: age, possible contacts, past ocular history, allergies or previous history of allergic conjunctivitis, make sure there is no pain involved for allergic and viral conjunctivitis.

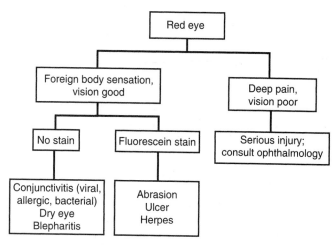

FIGURE 17-2. The red eye.

C. Symptoms:

Viral: Unilateral red eye, possible associated URI symptoms, mild itching, morning crusting or discharge.
Allergic: Bilateral itching, mild redness, watery discharge.
Bacterial: Acute purulent discharge, eyelid edema, decreased vision.

D. Physical exam:

Viral: Conjunctival injection, crusting, follicles.
Allergic: Lid swelling, chemosis, papillae.
Bacterial: Discharge.

E. Workup:

Bacterial: Gram stain and culture for *staphylococcus, streptococcus, H. flu, N. gonorrhea.*

F. Treatment:

Viral:

1. No specific medical treatment necessary—self-limited illness.

2. Symptomatic treatment with cool compresses or artificial tears.

3. Naphazoline (Naphcon A or Vasocon) may be prescribed tid × 7 days.

4. Wash hands, towels, pillowcases. Use separate towels. No contact lens wear for at least 7 days.

5. Avoid close contact (especially rubbing eyes and touching others) without washing hands first.

Allergic:

1. Eliminate inciting agent.

2. Cool compresses and artificial tears.

3. Olopatadine (Patanol) or nedocromil (Allocril) antihistamine drops bid.

Bacterial:

1. Bacitracin/polymyxin (Polysporin) ophthalmic ointment or erythromycin ointment qid.

2. For *H. flu*: Amoxicillin/clavulanate (Augmentin), 250–500 PO tid.

3. For GC: Ceftriaxone, 1 gm IM, and empiric treatment for chlamydia with azithromycin 1 gm PO × one. Treat sexual partners.

G. Clinical pearls: If vision is acutely and significantly reduced, a diagnosis of conjunctivitis is UNLIKELY. Any pupillary inequality in a patient with red eye(s) is a danger signal for serious ocular disease. Immediate ophthalmologic consultation is warranted in these situations.

Acute Hordeolum (*Stye*)

A. Not an emergency.

B. Symptoms: Pain, redness, "bump."

C. Physical exam: Red, tender, swollen nodule around the lid margin or hair follicle.

D. Treatment:

1. Hot compress to eyelids for 5 minutes, 5 times a day.

2. Empiric topical antibiotic such as bacitracin/polymixin (Polysporin) or erythromycin ophthalmic ointment tid.

3. Follow up with ophthalmologist in 1 week.

ORTHOPEDIC SURGERY
Fractures

A. *Open fractures and fractures with associated neurovascular compromise are emergencies—call a consult immediately!*

B. Pertinent history: mechanism of injury and preinjury level of activity.

C. Pertinent physical exam: complete distal neurologic and vascular exam.

D. Before calling an orthopedic consult for fracture, plain radiographs of the bone involved must be obtained. Usually AP and lateral views are sufficient. However, in certain instances additional views are necessary. The following list contains some common fractures in which additional views are necessary for diagnosis, preop planning, or both.

1. Shoulder/proximal humerus: AP, true AP, axillary view, scapular lateral (or Y) view.

2. Femoral neck/intertrochanteric fractures: AP hip, cross-table lateral, AP ortho pelvis.

3. Acetabular fractures: AP ortho pelvis, Judet views.

4. Ankle: AP, lateral, mortise.

5. Foot: AP, lateral, medial oblique; obtain a Harris heel (axial) view if a calcaneal fracture is suspected.

E. Describing fractures: Attempt to delineate the following:

1. Fracture pattern (transverse, oblique, spiral)

2. Displacement

3. Angulation

4. Shortening

5. Comminution

6. Open versus closed:

   • Open fractures are graded I–III, with III being most severe.

   • Grade I fractures have wounds less than 1 cm in length.

   • Grade II fractures have wounds greater than 1 cm.

   • Grade III fractures are subdivided as follows:

     IIIa: Wound >10 cm without periosteal stripping.
     IIIb: Periosteal stripping.
     IIIc: Associated vascular injury.

F. Workup: Usually plain radiographs are sufficient. However, if an occult fracture is suspected, obtain either an MRI or a bone scan to confirm. For hip fractures, bone scans may not be positive until 2–3 days postinjury. MRI will be positive within 24 hours.

G. Initial treatment/management:

1. Open fractures require emergent operative debridement and fixation.

2. Keep patients NPO.

3. Give tetanus toxoid.

4. Give IV antibiotics according to fracture grade.

   - Grade I fractures—cefazolin

   - Grade II fractures—cefazolin and gentamicin

   - Grade III fractures—cefazolin, gentamicin, and penicillin (if associated with gross soft tissue contamination)

5. Closed fractures are treated on an individual basis based on particular bone involvement and amount of displacement.

6. When lower extremity fractures are diagnosed, consider initiating DVT prophylaxis with antiembolism stockings and sequential compressive devices, subcutaneous LMWH, or both.

Septic Joint

A. *This is an **emergency**—call a consult immediately!*

B. Pertinent information: history and exam consistent with effusion, warmth, painful range of motion, tenderness, and fever.

C. Workup: plain radiographs, CBC, ESR, CRP, and blood cultures (if febrile). The diagnosis is confirmed with joint aspiration. Aspiration may be done by the primary physician or an orthopedics consultant. Synovial fluid should be sent for stat Gram stain, cell count, crystals, and culture. Antibiotics should not be administered until a joint aspirate is obtained. The patient should be made NPO until the cell count and Gram stain result are found to be negative for infection.

D. Diagnosis:

1. Septic arthritis is diagnosed with a synovial fluid leukocyte count generally >80,000 per cubic mm, a positive Gram stain, or a positive culture result.

2. An inflammatory/autoimmune arthropathy typically has a synovial fluid leukocyte count of 10,000–50,000 per cubic mm with positive crystals (for gout or CPPD disease), and negative Gram's stain and culture results.

E. Treatment:

1. Operative drainage. [*Neisseria* species (*gonorrhoeae* and *meningitidis*) are exceptions to this rule, as they are highly responsive to antibiotic therapy; operative debridement is not necessary.]

2. Appropriate intravenous antibiotics as determined by cultures. The course of antibiotics is typically 6 weeks total with the first 1–2 weeks being intravenous antibiotics.

3. Once the diagnosis is confirmed, the patient should be made NPO in preparation for operative drainage.

F. Clinical pearls: *S. aureus* is the most common orthopedic pathogen overall. In sexually active adolescents and adults, *N. gonorrhoeae* has a particularly high prevalence, whereas *Salmonella* has a particularly high prevalence in sickle cell patients.

Compartment Syndrome

A. *Compartment syndrome is an **emergency**—call a consult immediately!*

B. Definition: Compartment syndromes are caused by elevated hydrostatic pressure within a fascial compartment, leading to tissue ischemia as compartment pressure exceeds capillary pressure. Elevated hydrostatic pressure commonly occurs from bleeding or swelling from within the compartment.

C. When to consider this: The most specific signs and symptoms of compartment syndrome are pain out of proportion to injury, pain with passive stretch of the muscles in the involved compartment, and hard tense compartments. Paraesthesias, pallor, pulselessness, and paralysis may or may not be present. All external circumferential dressings should be removed before examining a patient for compartment syndrome.

Typical history may include the following:

1. Trauma (fracture or muscle contusion)

2. Ischemia

3. Venous obstruction

4. Massive inflammation from snake or insect bites

5. Bleeding into the compartment (consider in anticoagulated patients)

6. Infiltration of fluid material into a compartment (paint gun injuries)

7. Tight circumferential dressings

D. Diagnosis: The diagnosis is a clinical one. However, when clinical signs are equivocal, compartment pressures may be measured by an orthopedics consultant. Compartment pressures >30 mm Hg (or a diastolic blood pressure compartment pressure difference >30 mm Hg for hypotensive patients) are diagnostic for compartment syndrome.

E. Treatment:

1. Make patient NPO immediately.

2. Emergent fasciotomy.

F. Clinical pearls: Remember that myoglobinuria can occur with compartment syndrome from muscle necrosis.

Acute Cauda Equina Syndrome

A. *This is an **emergency**—call a consult immediately!*

B. Definition: Cauda equina syndrome is an injury to the spinal canal located between the conus and the lumbosacral nerve roots, resulting in bowel and bladder dysfunction, saddle anesthesia, severe lower extremity neurologic deficit, and anal sphincter laxity.

C. Pertinent history: Suspect in a patient with low back pain and the previously mentioned signs and symptoms.

D. Pertinent physical exam: A complete lower extremity neurologic exam should be performed including lower extremity strength, sensation, and reflexes. A rectal exam should also be performed to assess rectal tone and perianal sensation. Remember that the cauda equina functions as the peripheral nervous system. Therefore, in a complete cauda equina injury, all peripheral nerves to the bowel, bladder, perianal area, and lower extremities will be lost, resulting in absent bulbocavernosus, anal wink, and lower extremity reflexes.

E. Workup: Stat AP and lateral views of the lumbar spine and a stat MRI of the lumbar spine. If the patient has had a prior discectomy, obtain MRI with gadolinium contrast. If the patient has had previous spine instrumentation, obtain a CT myelogram.

F. Treatment:

1. Make patient NPO immediately.

2. Emergent operative decompression.

OTOLARYNGOLOGY
Airway Emergencies

A. *Call a consult or the airway pager immediately for assistance!*

B. Pertinent history: When did the stridor commence; how long has it persisted; is it constant or intermittent, and is it progressing and to what degree (the degree of stridor may not necessarily indicate the severity of obstruction)? History of prior intubation (and any previous difficulty); trauma; laryngeal surgery; or previous tracheostomy?

C. Pertinent physical exam: Cardinal sign of airway obstruction is stridor secondary to turbulence of air in the upper airways. Inspiratory stridor usually indicates partial supraglottic obstruction (i.e., trauma/fractures, foreign bodies, hematomas, edema). Expiratory stridor usually indicates glottic or subglottic pathology. Combined inspiratory and expiratory stridor suggests partial obstruction at the level of the glottis. Other signs of respiratory distress may include restlessness, drooling, suprasternal retractions, and hoarseness. A hoarse voice may mean laryngeal involvement. A muffled cry may mean supraglottic involvement. Coughing or choking may refer to vocal cord paralysis, aspiration, reflux, or an anatomic abnormality (laryngeal cleft or TE fistula).

D. Workup: Usually in a true airway emergency, there is no time for diagnostic tests until a stable airway is attained. Some diagnostic tests to evaluate respiratory distress include blood gas, CBC, CXR, soft tissue airway films (may demonstrate supraglottic edema/subcutaneous emphysema), CT scan of the neck, and C-spine films in cases of trauma.

E. Treatment:

1. Cool humidified room air or oxygen helps to prevent crust formation.

2. Oxygen per nasal cannula, face mask, nonrebreather.

3. Heliox refers to a 80%:20% helium-oxygen mixture. It relies on decreased density of helium to transport oxygen past the obstructive site.

4. Systemic corticosteroids may be used to acutely decrease edema from trauma/infectious etiology [dexamethasone (Decadron) or methylprednisolone (Solu-Medrol IV)].

5. Racemic epinephrine works quickly, acting as a topical decongestant; however, it is short-acting, and there may be a rebound effect once it dissipates.

F. Clinical pearls:

1. Nasopharyngeal airway is beneficial for patients emerging from general anesthesia or who have mild head trauma but normal respiratory drive. Nasopharyngeal trumpet can be used to open the airway when relaxation of soft palate/base of the tongue occurs.

2. Oropharyngeal airway may treat ventilatory obstruction due to a relaxed tongue.

3. Transoral intubation is the standard for airway control. **Contrain-dications** include C-spine fractures and laryngeal fractures.

4. Consultation is advised for possible fiberoptic intubation (in case of difficult intubation), airway distress refractory to therapeutic options, exam of supraglottis/glottis (i.e., rule out vocal cord paralysis, neoplasm, foreign body).

Tracheotomy

A. The optimal timing for a tracheotomy is controversial. Evaluation of the patient at 7–10 days after intubation is appropriate to assess for likelihood of extubation. If long-term intubation is probable, then a tracheotomy is justified. In some patients with neuromuscular disorders (i.e., Guillain-Barré syndrome) in which long-term ventilatory support is anticipated, earlier tracheotomy may be done.

B. Types: Shiley and Portex tracheostomy tubes are plastic and may be with or without cuffs. Both may be used initially after the surgical procedure. Typically, tracheostomy tubes are kept undisturbed for 3–5 days to allow formation of a well-healed tract. After this point, the plastic tracheostomy tubes are changed to a metal (Jackson) tracheostomy tube for long-term use or Shiley/Portex trach tubes (cuffed) if ventilatory support is still needed.

C. ENT will do the first tracheostomy change after 3–5 days to ensure a well-healed tract has formed. Frequent cleaning or changing of the inner cannula is recommended to prevent obstruction by crusting (typically at least tid).

- If the trach tube falls out, first assess whether the patient is breathing adequately through the stoma site.

- If the patient is stable and there is no one experienced in trach management, then call the surgical service for assistance.

- If the patient is not stable, then the trach tube usually can be reinserted *with the aid of the obturator.*

- If respirations are still difficult, then the tube is likely in a false tract. The correct tract may be found with the aid of a Kelly clamp to open the stoma site or by passing the trach tube over a fiberoptic scope, suction catheter, or Foley catheter.

- Transoral intubation is always an option.

Epistaxis Emergency

A. *Call a consult immediately for assistance!*

B. Pertinent history: airway status, history of trauma, anticoagulant medications, systemic diseases causing bleeding diatheses (e.g., hemophilia, liver disease, von Willebrand's disease, hereditary hemorrhagic telangiectasia).

C. Pertinent physical exam: Determine the source of bleeding (anterior versus posterior and right versus left nare). Identification of most anterior sites can be aided by nasal speculum and light source (headlight or mirror).

D. Workup: Check coagulation values including bleeding time and hematocrit. Check blood pressure, and treat hypertension.

E. Diagnosis: Bleeding from the nasopharynx or nares causing respiratory distress and aspiration.

F. Treatment:

1. Epistaxis tray at bedside: nasal speculum, 4% lidocaine, antibiotic/Vaseline-coated gauze for nasal packing, epistaxis anterior pack (Merocel), Surgicel, silver nitrate sticks, or Epistat (modified Foley balloon with pack) for posterior bleeding.

2. Application of topical vasoconstrictive agents [oxymetazoline hydrochloride (Afrin) 0.05%, phenylephrine hydrochloride 0.25%, or 4% cocaine] may slow down the bleeding.

Epistaxis Urgency

A. Call the ENT resident for an urgent consult.

B. Pertinent history: See previous section regarding pertinent history. Consider local factors including trauma, nasal sprays (decongestants and steroid nasal sprays), foreign bodies, anatomic deformities (septal perforations), nasal prong oxygen, local inflammation due to chronic sinusitis, allergic rhinitis, nutritional deficiencies, and alcohol abuse.

C. Diagnosis: Bleeding from the nasopharynx or nares refractory to *constant* nasal compression for 15–30 minutes at the nasal ala.

D. Treatment:

1. Keep patient seated instead of supine because of risk of choking or swallowing blood.

2. May be managed with selective use of silver nitrate stick if it is a well-visualized anterior bleed.

3. May require either Merocel anterior packing or Vaseline-coated gauze packing for 3–5 days.

4. May require Epistat if there is a posterior bleed refractory to anterior packing.

Epistaxis (General)

A. Clinical pearls:

1. Usually simple nasal compression for 15 minutes will stop the bleeding.

2. Control hypertension.

3. Nasal cannula prongs may irritate and dry the septal mucosa. Replace with humidified O_2 and frequent use of saline (Ocean) nasal spray.

4. Do not apply silver nitrate to adjoining sides of the septum. This may lead to a septal perforation.

5. All patients with nasal packing require antistaphylococcal antibiotic coverage to reduce chance of toxic shock syndrome.

6. The most common hereditary bleeding disorder associated with epistaxis is von Willebrand's disease.

Acute Sinusitis—Emergency

A. *This is an emergency when the infection has extended past the sinuses—call a consultant immediately!*

B. Pertinent history: duration of sinusitis symptoms, vision changes, mental status changes, duration of antibiotic therapy. Predisposing factors such as malnutrition, diabetes mellitus, chemotherapy, long-term corticosteroids, allergic rhinitis, immunodeficiency states, environmental exposures, and placement of NG tube.

C. Pertinent physical exam: meningeal signs and orbital signs (proptosis, chemosis, impeded extraocular movement, vision loss). These suggest extension of the infection beyond the sinus and necessitate immediate attention by an ENT consultant.

D. Workup: CT scan of sinus, high-resolution CT scan of orbits to rule out subperiosteal or orbital abscess.

E. Diagnosis: Clinically diagnosed sinusitis with evidence of extension to the intracranial area or orbits.

F. Treatment:

1. IV antibiotics (broad-spectrum).

2. Copious use of saline (Ocean) nasal spray and oxymetazoline (Afrin) to aid in nasal drainage.

3. IV steroids to help diminish edema around orbits and reduce optic nerve damage.

4. Surgery (functional endoscopic sinus surgery) is definitive therapy to drain abscess and sinuses.

5. If optic nerve damage is imminent, then lateral canthotomy with tendon cantholysis should be done to decrease intraocular pressure.

Vertigo

A. Vertigo emergency

1. *Important vertigo emergencies* include the following:

   a. Wallenberg's syndrome

   b. Lateral pontomedullary syndrome

   c. Cerebellar hemorrhage

   d. Cerebellar infarction

   e. Vertebrobasilar insufficiency

2. Pertinent history: Sensation and duration of dizziness, associated symptoms (especially neurologic symptoms), nausea, or vomiting.

3. Pertinent physical exam: Associated neurologic findings (diplopia, dysphasia, drop attacks, vision loss, dysphagia, loss of pain/temperature sensation, loss of motor control), Horner's syndrome, nuchal rigidity, papilledema, bidirectional gaze-fixation nystagmus, failure of gaze suppression nystagmus, spontaneous upbeat or downbeat nystagmus. Nylen-Bárány maneuver: Try to produce the vertigo and nystagmus by having a seated patient quickly lie down while turning his or her head to one side.

4. Workup: CT/MRI or cerebral angiogram (depending on etiology).

5. Diagnosis: By clinical exam and supporting imaging studies.

6. Treatment: Depending on etiology, may include surgical decompression, anticoagulation, and/or supportive care.

B. Vertigo (general)

1. Commonly seen etiologies by the otolaryngologist:

   a. Benign paroxysmal positional vertigo

   b. Ménière's disease

   c. Vestibular neuronitis

   d. Migraine-associated vertigo

2. Pertinent history: See Vertigo Emergency section. Also note exacerbating factors (especially sudden head motion), associated hearing loss, tinnitus, aural fullness, other otologic symptoms, general medical history, medications.

3. Pertinent physical exam: Nausea and vomiting (these tend to point to peripheral cause), horizontal nystagmus, fixation suppression of nystagmus, Nylen-Bárány maneuver (reproducible nystagmus and vertigo if seated patient turns head to one side while lying down quickly).

4. Workup: Rule out medical causes including hypotension or hypertension, cardiac arrhythmias, endocrine abnormalities.

5. Diagnosis: Mainly clinical diagnosis depending on duration, severity of symptoms, and physical exam.

6. Treatment:

   a. Compazine suppositories, 25 mg pr q6h.

   b. Meclizine (Antivert), 12.5–25 mg PO q8h prn.

   c. Diazepam (Valium), 2–10 mg PO q6h prn.

   d. For severe cases, diazepam, 5–10 mg IM or droperidol, 2.5 mg IM.

   e. In general, treatment depends on exact etiology (e.g., BPPV treatment involves Epley or particle repositioning maneuver).

PSYCHIATRY
Key Points

A. A patient's right to refuse a psychiatric consultation

1. Psychiatric consultation in and of itself may be stigmatizing.

2. Patients have the right to refuse consultation, *unless*

   a. There is concern about the patient being a danger to him- or herself or others.

   b. There is concern about the patient's decision-making capacity.

3. Clinical pearl: The patient should always be told that a psychiatric consultant is coming to see him or her.

Suicidality

A. When to suspect ideation: when the patient appears sad, depressed, or anxious, when there is a significant drug or alcohol history, when there is a history of domestic abuse, when psychosis is present.

B. Before calling the consult, obtain the following information:

1. Key history: age, gender, previous psychiatric treatment, suicide plan, presence of psychosis and command hallucinations, presence of anxiety, current meds, brief general medical history, and hospital course.

2. Key physical findings: Presence or absence of agitation, anxiety, overt psychosis.

C. Treatment:

1. Keep patient safe; get a sitter until directed otherwise by psychiatry.

2. Do not let a suicidal patient leave without clearance from psychiatry; once medical issues are resolved, the patient may require transfer to psychiatry, possibly against the patient's wishes.

D. Clinical pearls:

1. Suicidal ideation is a symptom, not a diagnosis; a full psychiatric interview is necessary to determine the cause and direct treatment.

2. Never be afraid to ask about the presence of suicidality; you will *not* give the patients ideas they didn't already have.

Violent Patients

A. Critical diagnostic question: Is delirium present (i.e., does the patient have a fluctuating level of consciousness with altered mental status)?

B. Before calling the consult, obtain the following information:

1. Key history: age, gender, onset of symptom, level of orientation, presence of psychosis, prior psychiatric treatment, current meds, brief medical history, and hospital course.

2. Key physical findings: Vital signs, overt psychosis, localized findings on neurologic exam.

C. Workup: directed at identifying the cause of the delirium; may include lytes, CBC, U/A, LFTs, CSF studies.

D. Treatment:

1. Protect the patient and staff; sedate the patient with antipsychotics (e.g., haloperidol IM in doses ranging from 0.5 mg in the frail and elderly to 5 mg in the younger and larger); use restraints if necessary.

2. Identify and treat the cause of the delirium.

3. Family members can help reorient delirious patients and lessen their violence. Dimly lit, quiet rooms help, as do glasses and hearing aids for those who need them.

E. Clinical pearls:

1. Common, less obvious causes of delirium are anticholinergic medications, benzodiazepines, undertreated pain, opiates, and ste-

roids. Offending medicines should be tapered or discontinued as much as possible.

2. Avoid using benzodiazepines for sedation in delirious patients unless the delirium is from alcohol or sedative withdrawal.

3. Do not put yourself in danger. Remove all possible items in the vicinity that could be used against you (e.g., stethoscope).

4. Have security with you.

5. Stand between the patient and an open door.

Competency

A. Definitions

1. *Competence* is technically a legal term. Only a judge can declare someone incompetent (and appoint a guardian, for example).

2. *Decision-making capacity* refers to the ability of patients to give informed consent to medical care; psychiatrists can often assist in the assessment of capacity.

B. Competency is an emergency or urgency as the patient typically requires emergent or urgent medical care for which the patient is unable or unwilling to give consent.

C. Before calling the consult, obtain the following information:

1. Key historical information: age, gender, proposed medical care and risks, benefits, and alternatives particular to the patient, medical history, current meds, presence of psychosis or depression, psychiatric history.

2. Key physical findings: presence or absence of agitation, anxiety, overt psychosis.

D. Demonstration of decision-making capacity requires all three of the following:

1. Understanding of medical situation and likely outcome of no treatment.

2. Understanding of risks and benefits of treatment options.

3. Ability to manipulate information rationally and give a rational explanation for preferred treatment.

E. Clinical pearls:

1. Many consults to psychiatry result from patients not being adequately informed of the proposed treatment's risks and benefits.

2. Presence of psychosis does not necessarily mean that a patient lacks capacity (e.g., belief that one is part of the intergalactic

guard may have no bearing on understanding the risks and benefits of cardiac catheterization).

3. Capacity is decision specific; one may have capacity to take IV meds but not PO if one believes that all of the pills are sprayed with a poison.

4. Capacity is time specific. Demonstrating capacity today is no guarantee that one will be able to demonstrate capacity tomorrow should mental status fluctuate.

5. Psychiatric consultation can only help with determining if a patient lacks capacity to make a decision; the consult will not tell you who the decision-maker should be if the patient lacks capacity.

Psychosis

A. Definition: *Psychosis* is a break with reality demonstrated by hallucinations, delusions, or bizarre behavior.

B. Psychosis itself is not a psychiatric emergency. The psychiatric consult can wait until the morning. On a medical/surgical floor, psychosis is often a symptom of delirium, which can be a medical emergency.

C. Critical diagnostic question: Is the patient delirious (i.e., does the patient have a fluctuating level of consciousness with altered mental status)? If so, see the section on the violent patient for further discussion of delirium.

D. Before calling the consult, obtain the following information:

1. Key history: age, gender, previous psychiatric treatment, nature of psychosis and symptom onset, presence of anxiety, current meds, brief general medical history and hospital course, presence of suicidal or homicidal ideas, presence of command hallucinations.

2. Key physical findings: Presence or absence of agitation, anxiety, thought disorder, bizarre behavior.

E. Clinical pearls:

1. Visual hallucinations usually result from delirium or intoxication.

2. Auditory hallucinations are the most common form in psychiatric disorders.

3. Olfactory and gustatory hallucinations are usually seen in the aura of a seizure.

4. Tactile hallucinations can result from drug withdrawal.

5. Psychosis is a symptom, not a diagnosis; a full psychiatric interview is necessary to determine the cause and direct treatment.

Domestic Violence, Rape, and Psychiatric Trauma

A. Legal reporting requirements:

1. Physicians in every state are **required** to break confidentiality and report *suspected* cases of child abuse to local authorities, usually called the Division of Family Services or Child Protective Services.

2. Many states also require that suspected elder abuse be reported.

3. There are no such legal requirements for spouse abuse.

B. Rape victims should be referred to obstetrics and gynecology for collection of evidence, treatment of physical trauma, evaluation of exposure to STDs, and referred for follow-up counseling.

C. Psychiatric consultation may help with the treatment of depression, anxiety, substance abuse, posttraumatic stress disorder, and personality disorders that are all commonly found in the victims of domestic violence and rape. Perpetrators of domestic violence also frequently have many of these problems.

D. Before calling the consult, make sure the patient is willing to see a psychiatrist. Include the following information:

1. Key history: age, gender, previous psychiatric treatment, nature of symptoms, presence of anxiety and depression, current meds, brief general medical history and hospital course, presence of suicidal or homicidal ideas.

2. Key physical findings: Presence or absence of agitation, anxiety, overt psychosis.

E. Diagnosis: Questions regarding domestic abuse should be asked as a routine part of the social history on every patient.

F. Treatment:

1. Should begin with referral to a specific domestic violence support program if one is available locally.

2. Will depend on the patient's individual symptoms.

3. Generally includes allowing the patient to tell and retell the story of the trauma in a safe, supportive environment so that the associated anxiety lessens over time.

G. Clinical pearls:

1. If in doubt, call protective services regarding child abuse for more guidance.

2. Patients rarely volunteer information on being a victim of domestic violence; the first step toward helping them is to ask.

Chemical Dependency

A. Minor alcohol withdrawal (see also Chap. 13)

1. Diagnosis:

a. Tremors, headache, nausea, sweating, and autonomic instability occurring approximately 12 hours after the last drink and lasting up to 5 days if untreated.

b. No hallucinations, seizures, or delirium.

2. Treatment:

a. Benzodiazepines (e.g., lorazepam 0.5–1 mg q6–8h or chlordiazepoxide 100 mg qid) given scheduled and prn to keep vital signs stable, with a gradual taper over approximately 4 days.

b. Frequent monitoring of vital signs.

c. Adequate hydration.

d. Adequate replacement of electrolytes, particularly potassium and magnesium, as needed.

e. Replacement of vitamins, especially vitamin C, folate, and thiamine.

f. Seizure prophylaxis in those with a history of seizure.

g. The patient should be encouraged to allow psychiatric consultation for diagnosis and treatment of a possible chemical dependency.

B. Major alcohol withdrawal (a.k.a. *rum fits* and DTs) (see also Chap. 13)

1. This should not result in a straight psychiatric consultation. Consultation with a med-psych service or internal medicine may be appropriate, and such consultation may be emergent.

2. Diagnosis:

a. See the criteria under minor alcohol withdrawal.

b. Between 3 days and 2 weeks after the last drink, minor withdrawal symptoms become accompanied by hallucinations, seizures, or delirium. Autonomic instability worsens.

3. Treatment:

a. Same as for minor alcohol withdrawal, but monitoring of vital signs and supportive treatment are even more important; severe cases may require transfer to the ICU.

b. Haloperidol added to the benzodiazepine can help treat hallucinosis.

c. The patient should be encouraged to allow psychiatric consultation for diagnosis and treatment of a possible chemical dependency.

C. Cocaine and opioid withdrawal

1. Diagnosis:

   a. In opioid withdrawal: nausea, muscle aches, rhinorrhea, diarrhea, piloerection, craving.

   b. In cocaine withdrawal: fatigue, agitation, increased appetite.

2. Treatment:

   a. While both conditions are unpleasant for the patient, they are rarely medically serious.

   b. Opioid withdrawal can be treated with clonidine, 0.1 mg PO tid or a methadone taper.

   c. The patient should be encouraged to allow psychiatric consultation for diagnosis and treatment of a possible chemical dependency.

D. Chemical dependency

1. Before calling the consult, make sure the patient is willing to see a psychiatrist. Include the following information:

   a. Key history: age, gender, previous psychiatric treatment, amount of use, route of use, withdrawal symptoms, presence of anxiety and depression, current meds, brief general medical history and hospital course, presence of suicidal or homicidal ideas, presence of psychosis.

   b. Key physical findings: Presence or absence of agitation, anxiety, overt psychosis, withdrawal signs.

2. Diagnosis: Questions regarding alcohol and substance use should be asked as a routine part of the social history on every patient.

   a. Criteria revolve around tolerance, withdrawal, and inability to control use.

   b. If two of the CAGE questions (listed here) are positive, the patient should be encouraged to allow psychiatric consultation for more definitive diagnosis. Other patients, of course, may also be appropriate for referral.

      i. Ever tried to *C*ut down?

      ii. Had others get *A*nnoyed?

      iii. Felt *G*uilty about drinking?

      iv. Had an *E*ye opener (morning drink) to avoid withdrawal?

3. Treatment:

  a. Support groups such as AA.

  b. Anticraving medication such as naltrexone, nalmefene, or ondansetron for alcoholism.

  c. Methadone maintenance (from specially licensed clinics) for severe opioid dependence.

  d. Psychotherapy aimed at relapse prevention.

  e. Treatment of comorbid depression and anxiety disorders.

4. Clinical pearls:

  a. Sedative withdrawal has the same clinical picture as alcohol withdrawal.

  b. The shorter the half-life of the benzodiazepine (e.g., alprazolam), the more likely withdrawal.

  c. Untreated DTs has a mortality of over 15%.

  d. Drug use often accompanies STDs, physical trauma, and other medical conditions.

GENERAL SURGERY
Key Points

1. Time-efficient communication is crucial. If the surgeon is abrupt, do not take personal offense.

2. Identify yourself and the patient that needs a consult, then clearly identify the question you need answered (i.e., "this is a patient with a pulseless and painful leg").

3. Give an indication of the urgency of the consult (i.e., stat, a few hours, or sometime today).

4. Identify which surgical attending is requested, and then present the crucial information for the problem.

5. If important radiographs have been obtained, state their location (i.e., do not keep them in your call room).

Hernia

A. *A strangulated hernia is a surgical emergency—call a consult immediately!*

An incarcerated hernia is not necessarily a surgical emergency. If the hernia is reducible, this is not an urgent consult.

B. Pertinent information: Location and duration of the hernia, scar overlying hernia, associated symptoms, and status (strangulated, incarcerated, or reducible), time of patient's last bowel movement, fever, leukocytosis, or erythema of the skin overlying the hernia. Is the patient immunocompromised?

C. Physical exam: Diagnosis of a hernia is made by examining the patient in a standing position with the patient performing Valsalva's maneuver or coughing. A mass that protrudes is a hernia until proven otherwise. A *reducible* hernia is one that can return through its fascial defect. An *incarcerated* hernia is one that is irreducible (impossible to push back through the fascial defect). A *strangulated* hernia is one in which the blood flow of the hernia's contents is compromised leading to necrosis of the contained structures. The signs of this are a fever, leukocytosis, hypotension, erythema of the overlying skin, or extreme pain with light palpation of the hernia.

D. Treatment:

1. Attempt to reduce an incarcerated nonstrangulated hernia that does not protrude inferior to the inguinal ligament.

2. Place the patient supine in Trendelenburg's position and slowly apply firm, constant, circular pressure with the palm of the hand to the hernia.

   a. If the hernia reduces, then perform an abdominal examination an hour later to prove that ischemic bowel was not reduced. Then, call a non-urgent consult.

   b. If the patient has abdominal pain and you suspect ischemic bowel from the hernia, then call surgery urgently.

3. Most hernias require an operation if the patient can tolerate the risks of anesthesia.

4. Trusses or binders are usually not effective in the treatment of hernias.

E. Clinical pearls: Hernias are classified both by anatomy and status. Over 75% of hernias occur in the inguinal region, 10% are incisional or ventral hernias, 3% are femoral, and the remainder are of unusual types. The location is of less concern than the status of the hernia. Not all incarcerated hernias are strangulating. A freely reducible hernia is an elective consult that generally can wait to be requested until the morning.

Ischemic Lower Extremity

A. *Ischemic extremity is an emergency—call a consult immediately!*

B. An ischemic extremity may be due to acute events (embolic disease) or chronic disease (atherosclerosis). The acute event is an emergency because perfusion must be reestablished within 6–8 hours. Unlike patients with chronic disease, these patients have not developed collateral circulation to supply the lower leg.

C. Pertinent information:

1. Suspected source: embolism (atrial fibrillation/arrhythmia, LV aneurysm, AAA, or popliteal aneurysm), or chronic disease (atherosclerosis).

2. Status of the vascular system: Has this patient had vascular surgery, (if so, where does the bypass start and end?), where are the scars, and who was his or her surgeon?

D. Physical exam:

1. Status of collateral flow: Palpate or doppler pulses in the femoral, popliteal, dorsalis pedis, and posterior tibial arteries. Be able to tell the consultant if there is a temperature difference in the extremities and at what level (foot, shin, thigh, or whole leg).

2. Severity of ischemia: The most sensitive test to determine if the foot is viable is to test for proprioception of the toes. This will diminish within 5 minutes of cessation of blood flow. Next, test motor function and light touch.

E. Treatment options:

1. Most patients are started on intravenous heparin therapy.

2. Possible interventions include surgical bypass, surgical or interventional radiographic thrombectomy, or locally delivered intravascular thrombolytics.

Ischemic Ulcer of the Lower Extremity

A. Ischemic ulcer of the lower extremity is an elective consult.

B. Pertinent information:

1. These ulcers are commonly found on the first metatarsal head or tips of the toes and are due to a combination of unrecognized trauma, poor circulation, and infection. These are distinguished from venous stasis ulcers by location (which are usually on the lower anterior shin), vascularity (heaped up, engorged edges), and sensitivity (very painful).

2. Status of the vascular system: Has this patient had vascular surgery (if so, where does the bypass start and end?), and/or where are the scars?

3. Have any ankle-arm indices been performed?

    4. Are there any radiographs that document osteomyelitis of the underlying bone? Any exposed bone is assumed to have osteomyelitis until proven otherwise.

C. Pertinent physical exam: Palpate or doppler pulses in the femoral, popliteal, dorsalis pedis, and posterior tibial arteries. Signs of infection (e.g., pus discharge with palpation).

D. Treatment options:

    1. Amputation, debridement, or any procedure to increase vascular inflow in arterial disease and promote wound healing.

    2. Leg elevation, Unna boots, or compression stockings to encourage venous drainage in venous disease.

Retroperitoneal Bleeding

A. Retroperitoneal bleeding is an urgent consult.

B. Retroperitoneal bleeding is most commonly seen in patients after coronary angiography and is partially due to the frequent use of anticoagulant and antiplatelet medications. The hallmark for diagnosis is a decreasing hematocrit in a patient complaining of flank, back, or abdominal pain.

C. Pertinent information: What procedure was performed? What anticoagulants and antiplatelet agents were used, and have they been stopped? How much and over what time period has the hematocrit decreased? On the CT scan (go see it yourself; do not trust the radiologist), how large is it (in centimeters)? Does it compress the urinary system causing hydronephrosis or hydroureter, or compress the renal vein? These last two findings may necessitate urgent percutaneous nephrostomy tubes or surgery, respectively.

D. Pertinent physical exam: Neurologic status of the patient's ipsilateral leg? Test this by asking the patient to straight leg lift and then test light touch on the medial and lateral upper thigh. If these senses are diminished, the patient may need urgent operative decompression of the hematoma.

E. Diagnosis: Abdominal CT scan secures the diagnosis.

F. Treatment options:

    1. Variable treatment depending on situation.

    2. Check CBC immediately and follow frequently thereafter.

    3. Reverse anticoagulation with vitamin K and FFP as needed.

    4. Supportive measures (fluids, blood) and/or operative intervention.

Femoral Artery Pseudoaneurysm

A. *Emergency consult if there is compression of the femoral nerve;* it is urgent in most other cases.

B. Pertinent information: This complication of arterial puncture occurs in the same patient population as retroperitoneal hemorrhages. What procedure was performed? What anticoagulants and antiplatelet agents were used, and have they been stopped? How large is the pseudoaneurysm by ultrasound and does it have a long, thin neck? These pseudoaneurysms are more likely to spontaneously thrombose or be amenable to ultrasound-guided compression.

C. Physical exam: The hallmark of diagnosis is a thrill or bruit over the puncture site. Is there any evidence of emboli to the ipsilateral foot. Look at the tips of the toes and search for petechiae or new larger purple or black spots. If present, the patient may need immediate operative intervention. Is there any evidence of compression of the femoral nerve? Test motor function and light touch sensation in the leg. If absent, the patient may need immediate operative intervention.

D. Diagnosis: Ultrasound secures the diagnosis.

E. Treatment options: vary from expectant management to ultrasonic compression or operative closure of the arteriotomy and evacuation of the hematoma.

Small Bowel Obstruction

A. Small bowel obstruction is an urgent consult. The most common causes are hernias, previous abdominal operations, and carcinoma.

B. Pertinent information: The hallmarks of diagnosis are abdominal distension, nausea, vomiting, waves of abdominal pain progressing to constant pain (an ominous sign), and cessation of bowel movements.

1. Which symptoms are present? How long have they been present?

2. When was the patient's last bowel movement?

3. Is the patient febrile (and do they have a leukocytosis)?

4. Are there any hernias?

5. Have they had any previous abdominal or pelvic operations?

6. What is the NG tube and Foley catheter output?

C. Physical exam: Check for hernias in the groin, umbilicus, and all scars for incisional hernias.

D. Diagnosis: What does the obstructive series show (do not order only a KUB), and is there colonic or rectal air? Most important, does the radiograph demonstrate any free air?

E. Treatment options:

1. Most patients without hernias who have not had previous abdominal operations will need to go to the operating room fairly soon.

2. In those that have had a previous abdominal operation:

    a. Make patient NPO.

    b. Nasogastric decompression.

    c. Fluid resuscitation.

    d. Frequent abdominal exams.

    e. Call surgery immediately if symptoms worsen.

F. Clinical pearls: The most common causes of SBO are hernias, previous abdominal operations, and carcinomas.

Hints for Diagnosis of an Acute Abdomen

An acute abdomen warrants immediate surgical intervention. These hints are not rigid rules because the diagnosis of an acute abdomen can require much judgment. The most common signs indicating an acute abdomen are peritoneal signs due to peritoneal inflammation.

... If there is any doubt at all, call ...

Signs:

- Rebound: This should never be tested for by pushing into the patient's abdomen and releasing. Not only is it barbaric but also not sensitive. Instead, pain with percussion on the anterior abdominal wall is the best test.

- Tussion: A patient who can cough several times probably does not have peritoneal signs.

- Laughing: A patient who laughs probably does not have peritoneal signs.

- Sitting up for posterior chest auscultation or rolling over for a rectal examination: Most patients with peritoneal signs will not do this.

Abdominal Pain with a Pulsatile Abdominal Mass

A. *Abdominal pain with a pulsatile abdominal mass is an incredible emergency!*

B. Abdominal pain with a pulsatile abdominal mass, suggesting a AAA, is the easiest problem you will ever evaluate:

1. Call surgery for a stat consult.

2. Type and cross the patient for six units of blood.

Pneumothorax

A. Pneumothorax is usually an urgent consult; it is an *emergent* consult if the patient is receiving positive pressure ventilation.

B. Pertinent information:

1. Which side?

2. Where is the CXR?

3. Is the patient on positive pressure ventilation? If so, this can be very dangerous and you must carefully monitor the patient until tube thoracostomy is performed. Get a chest tube tray and a 22 French chest tube to the bedside. If the patient decompensates, place a 14 or 16 angiocatheter in the second interspace at the midclavicular line of the affected side.

C. Treatment: Options vary as to the size and the physiologic impact of the pneumothorax:

1. Expectant management with serial chest radiographs may suffice in a young patient with negative pressure ventilation and no shortness of breath.

2. Needle aspiration of the air collection may be chosen.

3. Other patients may require open tube thoracostomy or percutaneous tube thoracostomy (a 14 French Thal tube).

Perirectal Abscess

A. Generally this is an urgent consult unless the patient is **septic**, then it is an *emergency*! Remember that there is no such thing as an unimportant abscess. It should always be evaluated by a surgeon.

B. Pertinent information: Is the patient diabetic or immunosuppressed? If so, then they are far more likely to die or have greater morbidity from this disease. Is the patient febrile, and do they have a leukocytosis?

C. Physical exam:

- Where is it (relative to the scrotum/vagina, and anus)?

- How far does the erythema and induration extend? If the stigmata of infection extends out from the anus, then the patient may have a Fournier's gangrene, which is a surgical emergency!

D. Treatment options:

1. Incision and drainage either at the bedside or in the operating room.

2. Fournier's gangrene will necessitate wide debridement in the operating room with massive irrigation of affected areas.

3. IV antibiotics.

E. Clinical pearls: "Perirectal abscess" is a misnomer. According to Park's classification system, there is no such thing as a perirectal abscess.

18

Guide to Procedures

... It's just a little sting, you won't feel a thing ...

TABLE 18-1.
ALL YOU REALLY NEED TO KNOW ABOUT VASCULAR ACCESS

Type	Description	Common Uses	Duration of Use
Triple-lumen catheter	3 separate lumens. Placed via the Seldinger technique usually at the bedside. Subclavian or internal jugular veins preferred, femoral vein can be used.	When peripheral access is exhausted and in emergency situations. Blood may be drawn from the catheter.	Short-term use (~7 days). Replace femoral lines more frequently (~3 days)
Hickman catheter	Surgically placed (single or multilumen). Subcutaneously tunneled. Dacron cuff at the skin entry site. Located in subclavian vein (tip is located near the right atrium).	Long-term intravenous medications and/or fluids. Blood may be drawn from the catheter.	Long-term use. May be left in place indefinitely as long as functioning properly.
Hohn catheter	Single- or doble-lumen Silastic catheters. Placed via Seldinger technique by interventional radiology or surgery *without* a subcutaneous tunnel. Antimicrobial cuff at the skin insertion site. Located in subclavian or internal jugular veins.	Placed when peripheral access is exhausted. Administration of medications and fluids (when double-lumen). Blood may be drawn from the catheter.	Intermediate-term use (up to 6 weeks).

(Continued)

TABLE 18-1.
ALL YOU REALLY NEED TO KNOW ABOUT VASCULAR ACCESS (Continued)

Type	Description	Common Uses	Duration of Use
Implanted venous access device (Port-A-Cath)	Placed subcutaneously by a surgeon or interventional radiology. Single or double lumen. Specialized right-angle needle is required to access the portal chamber. Located in subclavian vein; tip is located near the right atrium.	Long-term intravenous medications and/or fluids, especially chemotherapy. Blood may be drawn from the catheter.	Intended for indefinite use.
Tunneled cuffed catheters (ASH, Duraflow, Tesio, etc.)	Dual lumen sialastic catheters. Placed by intervential radiology. Can be placed in the internal jugular vein or subclavian vein.	Used fro hemodialysis. Do not use catheter for any other reason without checking with nephrologist.	Intermediate-term use to allow graft or fistula maturation, if patients refuse permanent access, or if graft or fistula is contraindicated.
Midline catheter	*Kink proof* material. Peripherally placed by trained nursing personnel. Located in antecubital vein. Consider the possibility of midline catheter placement early before potential peripheral vessels are damaged.	Intermediate-term intravenous medications are planned (e.g., a several week course of antibiotics). Not intended for TPN or chemotherapy. Blood drawing is discouraged (causes fibrin deposition at the tip and eventual catheter failure.	Intermediate-term use (1–6 weeks). Heparin flushing should be performed when the catheter is not being used for therapy at least twice a day.

(Continued)

TABLE 18-1.
ALL YOU REALLY NEED TO KNOW ABOUT VASCULAR
ACCESS (Continued)

Type	Description	Common Uses	Duration of Use
PICC	17-inch Silastic catheter placed by trained nursing personnel. Interventional radiology can place PICC lines under fluoroscopy if necessary. Located in basilic, cephalic, or median cubital vein.	Long-term intravenous medications are planned. TPN and more irritation medications provided the tip is in the superior vena cava. Blood may be drawn from the catheter.	Long-term use. May be left in place indefinitely as long as functioning properly.

Complication from catheter placement may include bleeding, pneumothorax, infection, and thrombosis. Clotted catheters may be opened with urokinase.

VENIPUNCTURE
Indications

- Obtain venous blood for laboratory testing.

Contraindications

- Cellulitis, phlebitis, or venous obstruction at the site of venipuncture.

- Lymphangitis of the arm.

- Venipuncture site proximal to a peripheral IV site.

- Presence of an A-V fistula or graft.

What to Tell the Patient

A sample of blood will be taken from a vein. There may be a minor amount of pain. Bruising does sometimes occur after venipuncture. Informed consent is not required.

Equipment

- Tourniquet.

- Gloves.

- Alcohol prep swab.

- Vacutainer hub and appropriate needle. A 20-gauge needle and an appropriate sized syringe may also be used.

- Needles smaller than 22-gauge should be avoided because of the increased risk of hemolysis.

- Appropriate specimen tubes, labeled.

- Gauze pad and bandage.

- Patient labels.

Procedure

1. Apply the tourniquet above the antecubital fossa. Be careful that it is not so tight as to be uncomfortable.

2. Select an appropriate vein for venipuncture (usually the most easily palpable).

3. Swab the area with the alcohol prep pad.

4. Apply traction to the skin below the proposed site with the nondominant hand.

5. Holding the syringe or vacutainer in the dominant hand, enter the skin at a 15- to 30-degree angle with the needle bevel up either directly above or along side the vein. Then carefully advance the needle into the vein.

6. Either apply gentle back pressure on the syringe or press the first collection tube onto the needle inside the vacutainer hub.

7. Collect the quantity of blood required and/or fill and mix all the collection tubes.

8. Remove the tourniquet, withdraw the needle, and apply pressure to the site.

9. Apply the bandage.

10. Dispose of the needle properly.

Complications

- Hematoma.

- Phlebitis.

FEMORAL VEIN PHLEBOTOMY

Indications

- Femoral vein phlebotomy may be performed when it is impossible or impractical (e.g., emergency situations) to obtain blood from the arm.

Contraindications

- Cellulitis or venous obstruction at the site of venipuncture.

- Femoral vascular prosthesis over the site of venipuncture.

- Anticoagulation or bleeding disorder (relative contraindication).

What to Tell the Patient

A sample of blood will be taken from a vein in the groin. There will be more pain than from a typical venipuncture. Hematoma formation is not uncommon. The patient should lie supine with the ipsilateral thigh slightly abducted and externally rotated. Informed consent is not required.

Equipment

- Gloves.

- Alcohol prep swabs.

- An 18- or 20-gauge $1\frac{1}{2}$-inch needle and an appropriate sized syringe may also be used. A vacutainer hub and needle may also be used.

- Appropriate specimen tubes, labeled.

- Gauze pad and bandage.

- Patient labels.

Anatomy

The structures of the groin lie in the following order from lateral to medial: femoral **n**erve, femoral **a**rtery, femoral **v**ein, **e**mpty space, and **l**ymphatics (**NAVEL**). The femoral vein is directly medial to the femoral artery. The femoral pulse is easily palpated in most patients (Fig. 18-1).

Procedure

1. Determine the approximate location of the femoral vein by palpating the femoral pulse below the inguinal ligament.

2. Cleanse the area.

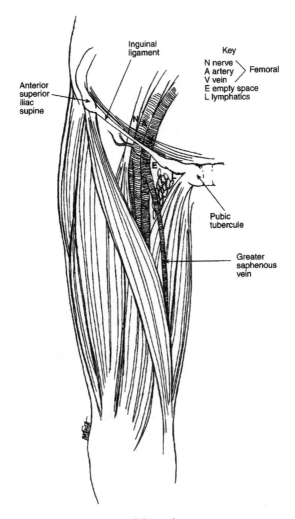

FIGURE 18-1. The structures of the groin.

3. Place the index and middle fingers of the nondominant hand over the femoral pulse (be careful not to contaminate the area just cleaned).

4. Holding the syringe or vacutainer in the dominant hand, insert the needle perpendicular to the skin just medial to the femoral artery.

5. Advance the needle slowly and smoothly while applying gentle back pressure. If there is no blood return and the needle is inserted to the hub, slowly withdraw the needle while continuing to apply gentle back pressure. If there is still no blood return, redirect the needle a bit more medially. If there is bright red blood return, the femoral artery has probably been entered. Go ahead and draw the blood that is required. Pressure will need to be applied for a longer duration.

6. Withdraw the appropriate amount of blood (or fill all specimen tubes).

7. Remove the needle and apply direct pressure with gauze for approximately 5 minutes.

8. Fill and mix the specimen tubes. An assistant is helpful at this point so that the phlebotomist can continue to hold pressure. In patients with a bleeding disorder, longer direct pressure is necessary.

9. Apply the bandage.

10. Dispose of the needle properly.

Complications

- Arterial puncture.

- Hematoma.

- Arteriovenous fistula (possible following repeated femoral phlebotomies on the same side).

PERIPHERAL IV

From time to time the house staff will be called on to place peripheral IVs. When you are asked, generally the nurse and IV therapist have been unsuccessful. Therefore, the IVs that you place will usually be fairly challenging.

Indications

- To gain peripheral intravenous access for the administration of fluids, medications, and/or blood.

Contraindications

- Cellulitis at the proposed site.

- Phlebitis or edema of the arm.

- Prior ipsilateral mastectomy or other axillary surgery in which venous drainage may be impaired.

- Presence of an A-V fistula or graft.

What to Tell the Patient

A small plastic catheter is going to be inserted into a vein in the hand or arm in order to give fluids and medications. There will be some minor pain with insertion. Patient cooperation is particularly important. Informed consent is not required.

Equipment

- Tourniquet.
- Gloves.
- Alcohol prep swabs.
- Povidone iodine prep swabs.
- IV fluids (saline flush).
- IV tubing.
- Appropriate catheter. A large gauge catheter must be used for infusion of viscous solutions such as blood and blood components (20-gauge or larger). For standard IV solutions and short-term infusions, a smaller catheter is acceptable (22-gauge). The smaller the catheter, the less the irritation to the vein.
- Occlusive dressing and tape.

Anatomy

Potential areas of insertion include the forearm, the dorsum of the hand, and the antecubital fossa. The most common sites are the veins of the hand, wrist, and forearm. The antecubital fossa should be avoided as bending of the elbow will disturb, occlude, and possibly dislodge the catheter. Always start at the most distal point of the extremity (e.g., the hand) if veins are present. Save the forearm and upper arm for later sites if possible. The lower extremities should *never* be used for IV placement.

Procedure

1. Assemble the fluids and tubing. Run fluid through the line, flushing all air, and recap the tubing.

2. Apply the tourniquet 4–6 inches above the proposed insertion site. Venous blood flow may also be occluded with a blood pressure cuff, but it should not obstruct arterial flow.

3. Select the vein to be used. Palpation is more important than visualization. Be sure the segment is long enough for the entire catheter.

4. Using a vigorous circular motion, prep the skin with alcohol. Allow to dry.

5. Using a circular motion, work from the center of the insertion site outward with the povidone iodine swab. Allow to dry.

6. Hold the skin taut and anchor the vein with the thumb of the non-dominant hand. Avoid recontamination of the insertion site.

7. Holding the catheter/needle assembly in the dominant hand, lower the hub of the needle close to the skin and align needle for insertion.

8. Insert the needle, bevel up, into the skin and subsequently into the vein. The skin may be punctured at the side of the vein or directly over it. In the side entry technique, the needle should puncture the skin on one side of the vein approximately $\frac{1}{2}$–1 inch below where the needle will enter the vein. Pierce the skin at a 45-degree angle along the side of the vein. Once through the skin, reduce the angle to approximately 20 degrees and enter the vein nearly parallel to the vessel. In the other technique, the skin should be punctured at a 45-degree angle directly over the vein. The angle is reduced to approximately 20 degrees and the vein is entered. If the needle is in the vein, blood return will be visible in the flashback chamber. Advance the needle a few more millimeters.

9. Release the tourniquet.

10. Carefully withdraw the needle approximately $\frac{1}{2}$ inch while continuing to advance the catheter. Apply pressure to the vein just above the tip of the catheter to obstruct blood flow. Remove the needle. *Never* reinsert the needle or pull the catheter back over the needle as this can shear off the plastic tip.

11. Connect the IV tubing to the catheter. To be certain the catheter is in the vein, lower the infusion bag below the level of the insertion site or gently aspirate with a 10 cc syringe filled with saline flush. Blood should appear in the tubing.

12. Cover the insertion site with a transparent occlusive dressing and tape securely.

Complications

- Hematoma.

- Phlebitis.

- Cellulitis.

- Sepsis.

- Extravasation of fluids and/or medications.

BLOOD CULTURES
Indications

- Documentation of bacteremia.

Contraindications

- Similar to those listed under venipuncture.

What to Tell the Patient

Two separate samples of blood are going to be collected for testing and two different needle sticks at two different sites will be required. Informed consent is not required.

Equipment

- Venipuncture supplies (previously listed).
- Sterile gloves.
- Alcohol prep swab sticks.
- Povidone iodine prep swab sticks.
- Blood culture bottles.
- Patient labels.

Procedure

1. Apply the tourniquet and select a venipuncture site. Release the tourniquet.

2. Vigorously cleanse the skin with three alcohol swab sticks. Work from the proposed puncture site outwards.

3. Swab the area concentrically with three povidone iodine swab sticks. Allow the skin to air dry.

4. Replace the tourniquet.

5. Do not touch the site unless wearing sterile gloves.

6. Perform the venipuncture and collect 20 cc of blood.

7. Without changing the needle, distribute 10 cc of blood to each of the culture bottles. Changing the needle may serve as a source of contamination. Gently mix the contents of the bottle.

8. Label each specimen bottle. The label should also have the drawer's initials, date and time, the word "blood" and the site (e.g., L arm). The specimen may be rejected if it is not properly labeled. Apply direct pressure with gauze over the puncture site and cover with bandage.

9. In almost all instances, you will obtain a second "set" of blood cultures from another site. If you must obtain the second set from the same site, wait approximately 5 minutes and follow the same disinfecting procedures *again*.

Complications

- Hematoma.

- Phlebitis.

ARTERIAL BLOOD GAS SAMPLING
Indications

- To obtain arterial blood for determination of blood gases.

Contraindications

- No palpable radial pulse (the preferred site, followed by the femoral then the brachial arteries).

- Poor collateral circulation in the hand (positive Allen's test).

- Cellulitis over the radial artery.

- Anticoagulation or bleeding disorder (relative contraindication).

What to Tell the Patient

A sample of blood is going to be obtained for testing from an artery in the wrist. It can be quite painful compared to venipuncture. Patient cooperation is particularly important. Informed consent is not required.

Equipment

- Gloves.

- Alcohol prep swab.

- ABG kit. If a kit is not available, a 3- to 5-cc syringe with a 23- to 25-gauge needle may also be used. The syringe should be heparinized by drawing up 0.5–1 cc of 1:1,000 heparin. Pull the plunger all the way back and then expel all the heparin.

- Ice in a cup or plastic bag.

- Gauze pad and bandage.

- Patient labels.

Procedure

1. Palpate the radial artery. Perform an Allen's test. Ask the patient to make a tight fist. Occlude the radial and ulnar arteries at the wrist. Have the patient relax the hand. Release the ulnar artery only. The hand should flush red in 5–6 seconds. If color return is delayed, there may be poor collateral flow, and a radial artery puncture should not be done on that side.

2. For femoral artery puncture, palpate the femoral pulse just below the inguinal ligament. Remember the mnemonic "NAVEL" (refer to Fig. 18-1).

3. Carefully palpate the chosen artery to determine where pulsations are the most prominent.

4. Swab the area with the alcohol prep pad.

5. Hold the syringe like a pencil. Point the needle proximally with the bevel up. Enter the skin at a 60- to 90-degree angle. Advance slowly until there is a flash of blood. If no flash is encountered, slowly withdraw the needle and continue to look for the flash.

6. Gently aspirate 1–2 cc of blood. The syringe may fill on its own.

7. Quickly remove the needle and apply firm pressure for 5 minutes.

8. Expel any air from the top of the syringe. Roll the syringe gently to mix so that it does not clot.

9. Dispose of the needle properly and cap the syringe.

10. Label the syringe and put it on ice.

11. Be sure the specimen gets to the lab as soon as possible.

Complications

- Hematoma.

- Infection.

- Thrombosis of the radial artery; ischemia of the hand.

CENTRAL VENOUS ACCESS

The most common sites for a central line are the right internal jugular vein, the subclavian veins, and the femoral veins. The usual method of obtaining central venous access is the over-the-wire technique (Seldinger's technique). The vein is first entered with a needle. A guidewire is passed through this needle. The needle is then withdrawn. The vessel is dilated. The catheter is then fed into the vein over the wire. **The most crucial part of the procedure is keeping hold of the guidewire. Never, ever let go of it.** (*Do you really want to be forever known as the intern that let go of the wire?*) It will be assumed that triple lumen catheter kits that contain most of the necessary equipment (e.g., catheter, wire, dilator, needles, suture, anesthetic, etc.) are available.

Indications

- Emergency venous access.

- Exhausted peripheral access.

- Rapid large volume fluid administration.

- TPN administration.

- Administration of multiple incompatible intravenous medications.

Contraindications

- Thrombosis of the selected vein.

- Unexplained edema of the face and/or associated arm or leg.

- Infection or cellulitis over the proposed site.

- Previous surgery in the proposed area.

- Anticoagulation or bleeding disorder (relative contraindication).

What to Tell the Patient

A large catheter will be placed in a large vein in order to provide better care. There are risks (see the following). The patient will experience some pain with the procedure. Positioning and cooperation are critical and should be explained to the patient in advance. **Informed consent is required.**

Equipment

- Sterile gloves.

- Appropriate materials to cleanse the skin (if not included in the kit).

- Gown, mask, goggles.

- Sterile drapes (if not included in the kit or if you want extra, which is always a good idea).

- Extra syringes, local anesthetic, and saline flush (just in case).

- Small syringes with normal saline to flush the catheter lumens after insertion.

- Triple lumen catheter kit.

Anatomy

- The internal jugular vein runs medial to the upper portion of the sternocleidomastoid muscle, deep to the triangle formed by the two heads of the mid-portion of the muscle, and then joins with the subclavian vein. The carotid artery is medial to the internal jugular vein (Fig. 18-2).

- The subclavian vein travels under the clavicle near apex of the lung. The subclavian artery is above and behind the vein (see Fig. 18-4).

- See Fig. 18-1 for the anatomy of the structures in the inguinal region.

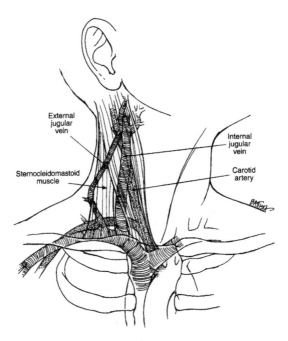

FIGURE 18-2. Central venous access.

Procedure

*Right Internal Jugular Vein (**Central Approach**)*

1. Obtain informed consent.

2. Enlist someone else to be your nonsterile assistant.

3. Place the patient in the Trendelenburg position. Have the patient turn his/her head to the left approximately 45 degrees.

4. Don goggles, mask, gown, and gloves.

5. Cleanse the site.

6. Drape the field.

7. Identify the apex of the triangle formed by the heads of the sternocleidomastoid muscle and also the carotid artery (refer to Fig. 18-2). Alternatively, portable ultrasound (e.g., Site Rite) can be used to localize the vein.

191

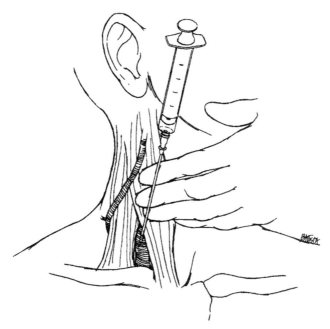

FIGURE 18-3. Accessing the right internal jugular vein (central approach).

8. Anesthetize the area.

9. Using a 22-gauge 2-inch needle and syringe, bevel up, at about a 30- to 45-degree angle to the plane of the patient, directed to the ipsilateral nipple attempt to locate the vein. Palpate the carotid artery with the nondominant hand as you go. The vein is usually encountered between 2–4 cm but can be more superficial. If unsuccessful, slowly withdraw the needle while aspirating. If there is still no venous blood return, redirect the needle slightly more laterally and then slightly more medially (*keep your fingers on the carotid artery*) while applying back pressure. If still unsuccessful, critically reassess the landmarks and patient positioning (Fig. 18-3).

10. If the carotid artery is inadvertently entered (bright red pulsatile blood that fills the syringe without back pressure), remove the needle and apply direct pressure for 10–15 minutes.

11. When venous blood is obtained, memorize the site and angle. Withdraw the needle.

12. Reinsert the large introducer needle supplied with the kit into the same site at the same angle until venous blood freely flows into the syringe again.

13. Securely hold the needle and remove the syringe. Always keep a finger over the open end of the needle to help reduce the risk of air embolization.

14. Gently pass the guidewire through the needle. It should advance easily without resistance. If resistance is met, remove the wire and check the needle placement again by replacing the syringe and withdrawing blood. Attempt to reintroduce the guidewire.

15. Leave enough of the guidewire outside the patient to accommodate the length of the catheter.

16. **While holding the guidewire's distal end,** remove the introducer needle from the patient. Now **hold the wire where it exits the skin** and slide the needle completely off the wire.

17. Nick the skin with a scalpel to enlarge the puncture site.

18. Thread the dilator onto the guidewire and gently into the vein. Remove the dilator. **Never lose hold of the guidewire.**

19. Thread the catheter onto the guidewire. **Do not pass the catheter into the vein until you have a firm hold on the distal end of the guidewire.** Pass the catheter into the vein **while continuously holding the distal end of the guidewire.** Open the distal port to accommodate distal end of guidewire.

20. While holding the catheter in place, remove the guidewire.

21. Confirm placement by withdrawing venous blood from all ports. Flush the ports.

22. Securely suture the catheter in place.

23. Apply povidone iodine ointment and an occlusive dressing.

24. Start IV fluids at a minimal rate.

25. Obtain a stat CXR to confirm the location of the catheter (tip should be in the SVC near the right atrium) and rule out pneumothorax.

26. Write a procedure note, whether or not you were successful.

Subclavian Vein

1. Follow steps 1 and 2 above for right internal jugular placement.

2. Patient positioning is especially important for successful subclavian placement. Place the patient in the Trendelenburg position. Place a

towel roll between the scapulae and allow the shoulder to fall back-wards. Both arms should be extended at the patient's sides. If the catheter will be inserted on the left (preferred), turn the patient's head to the right. If working on the right, turn the head to the left.

3. Follow previous steps 4, 5, and 6.

4. Place the index finger of the nondominant hand at the sternal notch. Place the thumb of the same hand at the point where the clavicle bends over the first rib (approximately the junction of the lateral one-third and the medial two-thirds of the length of the clavicle). The subclavian vein should traverse a line between the thumb and index finger (Fig. 18-4).

5. With a small gauge needle, anesthetize the skin and subcutaneous tissue just below the clavicle and lateral to the thumb.

6. Enter the skin with the introducer needle with the bevel facing up, lateral to the thumb and just caudal to the clavicle. While aspirating, slowly advance the needle under the clavicle toward the index finger parallel to the floor at all times. You may need to depress the needle

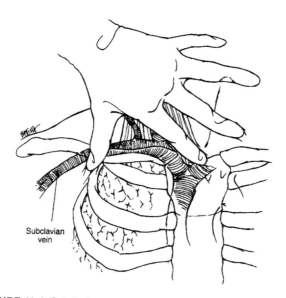

Subclavian vein

FIGURE 18-4. Subclavian vein should traverse a line between the thumb and index finger.

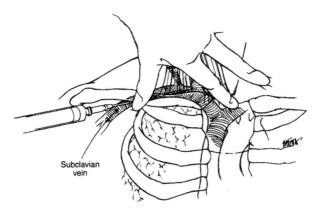

FIGURE 18-5. When the needle enters the subclavian vein there should be free return of dark blood.

with your thumb to get under the clavicle. When the needle enters the vein, there should be free return of dark blood. If there is no blood return after 5 cm, slowly withdraw the needle while continuing to aspirate. If there is still no blood return, redirect the needle to slightly above the sternal notch. Multiple attempts to redirect the needle are inadvisable (Fig. 18-5).

7. Once there is good venous return, rotate the syringe and needle so that the bevel is toward the feet.

8. Follow previous steps 14 through 27. If there is resistance to guidewire passage after it has cleared the tip of the needle, it may be going upward into the internal jugular vein. Remove the guidewire. Reconfirm the location of the needle by replacing the syringe and withdrawing venous blood. Turn the patient's head toward you and gently try to pass the guidewire again. Introduce the dilator only approximately 3–4 cm.

Femoral Vein

1. Obtain informed consent and enlist someone else to be your nonsterile assistant.

2. Place the patient in the supine position with the ipsilateral thigh slightly abducted and externally rotated.

3. Follow steps 4, 5, and 6 under Right Internal Jugular Placement.

4. Determine the approximate location of the femoral vein by palpating the femoral pulse below the inguinal ligament, using the "NAVEL" mnemonic (see Fig. 18-1).

5. Anesthetize the area with a small gauge needle. Be sure to aspirate before injecting.

6. While palpating the femoral artery, enter the skin below the inguinal crease and approximately 1 cm medial to the pulse with the introducer needle attached to a syringe at an approximate 30- to 45- degree angle, directed cephalad, and bevel up. While applying back pressure, advance the needle slowly and smoothly until there is free return of venous blood (Fig. 18-6). If there is no return after approximately 5 cm, slowly withdraw the needle while continuing to aspirate. If there is still no return, redirect the needle slightly more lateral. If there is return of arterial blood, withdraw the needle and hold firm pressure for approximately 10–15 minutes.

7. Follow steps 14 through 24 and 27 under Right Internal Jugular Placement once there is good venous return.

8. Be very cautious about advancing the guidewire in patients with an IVC filter—the IVC filter can be dislodged by the guidewire.

Complications

- Inadvertent arterial puncture.

- Pneumothorax.

- Hemothorax/hydrothorax.

- Retroperitoneal bleeding.

- Cardiac tamponade.

- Air embolus.

- Hematoma.

- Cellulitis.

- Line sepsis (most common with femoral lines).

- Thrombosis/embolism.

- Inadvertant dislodgment of IVC filter with the guidewire.

ARTERIAL LINE PLACEMENT

The preferred site for arterial cannulation is the radial artery. The technique can be difficult even for the experienced operator. The femoral artery is an alternative site.

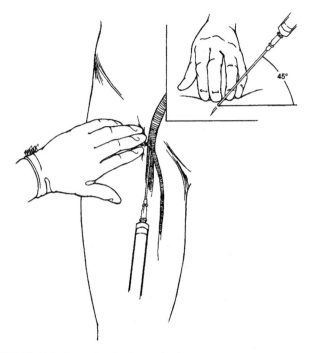

FIGURE 18-6. Accessing the femoral vein.

Indications

- Continuous arterial pressure monitoring.

- Frequent blood gas monitoring.

Contraindications

- Poor collateral circulation of the hand (e.g., failed Allen's test).

- Prior vascular bypass surgery, aneurysm, or severe atherosclerosis of the femoral artery.

- Anticoagulation or bleeding disorder (relative contraindication).

- Cellulitis over the proposed site.

- A-V fistula or graft in arm.

What to Tell the Patient

A catheter will be placed into an artery in the wrist or the groin in order to monitor blood pressure and/or to obtain frequent arterial blood samples. The procedure can be quite painful. **Informed consent** is required.

Equipment

• Sterile gloves.

• Appropriate materials to cleanse the skin (if not included in the kit).

• Gown, mask, goggles.

• Sterile drapes.

• Gauze sponges.

• Arm board and tape (radial artery only).

• Pressure infusion bag, pressure tubing, dilute heparin flush, appropriate transducer, and monitor (the ICU nurse will almost always know exactly what this entails and get it set up for you in advance so be sure to let him/her know that you plan to place an arterial line).

• Local anesthetic and small needles and syringes for administration.

• 20-gauge $1\frac{1}{2}$–2-inch Angiocath or quick catheter (radial artery) or 18-gauge introducer needle, guidewire, and 16-gauge, 6-inch arterial catheter (femoral artery).

• Suture.

• Sterile occlusive dressing.

Procedure

Radial Artery

1. Obtain informed consent.

2. Enlist someone else to be your nonsterile assistant (the ICU nurse is a good idea, as he or she will need to connect the line to the transducer and the transducer to the monitor).

3. Perform the Allen's test on the proposed side. Proceed only if there is good collateral flow.

4. Dorsiflex the patient's wrist and place a towel or gauze roll underneath. Secure the palm and forearm to an arm board with tape.

5. Don goggles, mask, gown, and gloves.

6. Cleanse the site.

7. Drape the field.

8. Carefully palpate the radial artery. Administer local anesthetic to the skin and subcutaneous tissue in this area. Be sure to aspirate before and injecting and do not aim directly for the artery.

9. Puncture the skin at a 45-degree angle with the 20-gauge Angiocath, pointing proximal, bevel up. Slowly and smoothly advance the catheter and needle (Fig. 18-7). When the artery is punctured, there will be a flash of bright red blood into the hub. If there is no flash, withdraw slowly and continue to watch for the flash. If there is still no flash, redirect toward the point of maximal pulsation again and advance carefully at a slightly steeper angle.

10. Once the Angiocath is in the arterial lumen, reduce the angle to approximately 20–30 degrees and advance the needle and catheter slightly (1–2 mm). Carefully slide the catheter off the needle into the lumen. If you are using a quick catheter, advance the guidewire into the artery and then pass the catheter over it. The catheter should pass without resistance. Remove the needle. Either occlude the artery proximally or be ready to put your finger over the catheter opening to prevent the forcible flow of arterial blood.

11. Immediately connect to the pressure tubing. There should be an arterial waveform on the monitor.

12. Suture the catheter in place.

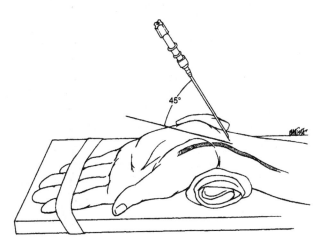

FIGURE 18-7. Accessing the radial artery.

13. Apply the dressing.

14. Write a procedure note, whether or not you were successful.

Femoral Artery

1. Follow steps 1 and 2 above for radial artery cannulation.

2. Place the patient in the supine position with the ipsilateral leg slightly abducted and externally rotated.

3. Locate the point of maximal femoral artery pulsation below the inguinal ligament using the "NAVEL" mnemonic (see Fig. 18-1).

4. Follow previous steps 5, 6, and 7.

5. Anesthetize the skin and subcutaneous tissue over the femoral artery (aspirate before injecting).

6. Using the 18-gauge introducer needle bevel up, puncture the skin at a 45-degree angle over the femoral pulsations. Advance the needle cephalad while continually aspirating. When the femoral artery is entered, there should be rapid return of pulsatile bright red blood. If there is no arterial blood after 5 cm, slowly withdraw the needle while aspirating. If there is still no blood return, redirect the needle toward the maximal pulsations and advance again.

7. When the artery is entered, remove the syringe from the introducer needle (be careful to occlude the pulsatile flow of blood with your finger).

8. Advance the guidewire into the artery. It should pass without resistance.

9. **While holding the guidewire's distal end,** remove the introducer needle from the patient. Now **hold the wire where it exits the skin** and slide the needle completely off the wire.

10. Make a small nick in the skin with a scalpel where the wire exits.

11. Thread the catheter onto the guidewire. **Do not pass the catheter into the artery until you have a firm hold on the distal end of the guidewire.** Pass the catheter into the artery **while continuously holding the distal end of the guidewire.**

12. Remove the guidewire and quickly place a finger over the open end of the catheter.

13. Follow previous steps 11 through 14.

Complications

- Thrombosis of the artery.

- Embolization of air, clot, or atherosclerotic material.

- Hematoma/hemorrhage.

- Retroperitoneal bleeding.

- Arteriovenous fistula formation.

- Pseudoaneurysm formation.

- Ischemia of the supplied area.

- Cellulitis, thrombophlebitis, sepsis.

LUMBAR PUNCTURE
Indications

- Analysis of CSF for diagnostic purposes.

- Injection of various agents into the CSF (e.g., contrast agent, antibiotics, chemotherapeutic agents).

- Drainage of CSF.

Contraindications

- Known or suspected intracranial mass and/or increased pressure.

- Infection over the site.

- Anticoagulation, bleeding disorder, or platelets <50K.

What to Tell the Patient

"Spinal taps" are associated with many myths. The procedure is associated with less pain and much less risk than the patient probably imagines. Proper positioning is critical, and you should enlist the patient's assistance with this. **Informed consent is required.**

Anatomy

In adults, the spinal cord usually terminates between L1 and L2. When a lumbar puncture is done, the goal is to obtain fluid from the lumbar cistern below this level. The puncture may be done at the L3/L4, L4/L5 (most common), or L5/S1 interspaces. The line connecting the posterior superior iliac crests (the intercristal line) intersects the spine at either the L4 spinous process or the L4/L5 interspace.

Equipment

- Sterile lumbar puncture kit.

- Extra small gauge needles, syringes, and local anesthetic (just in case).

- Appropriate materials to cleanse the skin (if not included in the kit).

- Sterile gloves.

- Mask and goggles.

Procedure

1. Obtain informed consent.

2. Enlist someone else to be your nonsterile assistant (not always necessary but nice to have around).

3. Place the patient in the lateral decubitus position with his or her back close to the edge of the bed or table. The patient should bring the knees up to the abdomen and flex the head to the chest as much as possible. The patient may need assistance holding this position (an assistant is very handy for this purpose). The procedure may also be done with the patient sitting and leaning forward. Obesity, osteoarthritis, and prior lumbar spine surgery may make positioning, identification of landmarks, and successful completion of the procedure very difficult.

4. Palpate the area of the intercristal line. Locate and mark the L4/L5 interspace.

5. Put on sterile gloves.

6. Cleanse the area and drape the patient.

7. Anesthetize the skin with a 25-gauge needle. Anesthetize to deeper structures with a 22-gauge needle.

8. Puncture the skin with spinal needle (stylet in place), bevel towards the head (parallel to the body's long axis). Carefully advance the needle between the vertebrae, aiming the tip cephalad at approximately 15–30 degrees (towards the navel), parallel to the floor. A ''pop'' will often be felt when the subarachnoid space is entered. Remove the stylet and observe for the flow of CSF. It may help to rotate the needle slightly. If there is none, replace the stylet (always be sure to do this) and advance a bit further. Remove the stylet again and so forth. If bone is encountered, pull back 1–2 cm and redirect.

9. When CSF flow is established, attach a manometer and stopcock. Measure the opening pressure (normal 70–180 mm). Collect ap-

proximately 3–4 cc of CSF in each tube. If cytology or other studies are to be done, more can be collected.

10. Replace the stylet and withdraw the needle.

11. Place a bandage over the site.

12. Write a procedure note, whether or not you were successful.

13. Instruct the patient to remain recumbent for 4–6 hours.

14. **Send the tubes** as follows: (1) Gram's stain, culture, AFB, fungal stain and culture; (2) glucose and protein; (3) CBC with differential; and (4) special studies as indicated. Refer to the Neurology section (Chap. 17, Table 17-1) for interpretation of CSF studies.

Complications

- Spinal headache.

- Trauma to the nerve roots.

- Herniation.

- Bleeding into the subdural or subarachnoid space.

- Meningitis.

THORACENTESIS
Indications

- Obtain pleural fluid for diagnostic testing.

- Drainage of pleural fluid in patients with large symptomatic effusions.

Contraindications

- Anticoagulation or bleeding disorder (relative).

- Severely impaired respiratory reserve to the degree that a pneumothorax could not be tolerated (relative).

What to Tell the Patient

A needle will be inserted through the chest wall to obtain pleural fluid for diagnosis and/or relief of symptoms. Pain is usually mild. Holding still is very important to reduce the risk of pneumothorax. **Informed consent is required.**

Anatomy

At least 250–300 cc of pleural fluid will be evident as blunting of the costophrenic angle on CXR. Pleural fluid may be loculated, and a decubitus film should be done to determine if the effusion is free flowing and large enough to attempt thoracentesis (usually >1 cm on lateral film). The intercostal vein, artery, and nerve travel in a groove along the inferior margin of the rib. Therefore, the entry site should be at the superior aspect of the rib.

Equipment

- Sterile thoracentesis kit.
- Extra small gauge needles, syringes, and local anesthetic (just in case).
- Appropriate materials to cleanse the skin (if not included in the kit).
- Sterile gloves.
- Mask and goggles.

Procedure

1. Obtain informed consent.

2. Enlist someone else to be your nonsterile assistant (not always necessary but nice to have around).

3. Have the patient sit on the edge of the bed leaning forward slightly on a bedside table. Percuss the location of the effusion and mark where the procedure will be attempted on the posterolateral chest.

4. Put on sterile gloves.

5. Cleanse the area and drape the patient.

6. Anesthetize the skin with a 25-gauge needle. Anesthetize to deeper structures including the rib periosteum with a 22-gauge needle.

7. Carefully advance the needle **over the superior aspect of the rib.** Continue to advance slowly until pleural fluid is aspirated.

8. Note the depth and trajectory. Remove the needle.

9. Make a small superficial nick in the skin at the needle entry site (to facilitate easy entry of the catheter/needle assembly).

10. Follow the same path with the catheter/needle assembly (attached to a syringe), aspirating all the way. Be sure to step over the rib.

11. When pleural fluid is obtained, slide the catheter into the pleural space and withdraw the needle. Place a finger over the opening of the catheter. **Never advance the needle back into the catheter.**

12. Attach a 30- to 50-cc syringe with a three-way stopcock to the catheter.

13. Attach connecting tubing to the sidearm of the stopcock. This may be connected to vacuum bottles or a collection bag. Pump out or allow the vacuum to suck out up to 1 L of pleural fluid. Do not

collect more than 1 L as this increases the risk of re-expansion pulmonary edema.

14. When finished collecting pleural fluid, have the patient hum or Valsalva and remove the catheter.

15. Bandage the site.

16. Write a procedure note, whether or not you were successful.

17. Obtain a CXR to rule out pneumothorax.

18. **Send pleural fluid** for cell count and differential, Gram's stain, routine culture, fungal stain and culture, specific gravity, protein, LDH, and glucose. If pH will be ordered, the sample must be fresh, in a heparinized syringe, on ice, and taken directly to the lab. Other tests may be done depending on the clinical situation. Refer to Table 18-2 regarding the interpretation of pleural fluid studies.

TABLE 18-2.
PLEURAL FLUID ANALYSIS

Parameter	Transudate*	Exudate**
Specific gravity	<1.016	>1.016
TP (g/dL)	<3.0	>3.0
Effusion TP/serum TP	<0.5	>0.5
LDH (IU)	<200	>200 (or >⅔ upper limit of normal)
Effusion LDH/serum LDH	<0.6	>0.6
Cholesterol	<45	>45
Glucose		Decreased in RA, cancer, TB, and empyema.
pH	~7.4	<7.3 suggests TB, malignancy, empyema, or RA; <7.2 suggests need for chest tube.
Cells	<1,000 WBC	>1,000 WBC
	<10,000 RBC	>10,000 RBC

* CHF, cirrhosis, nephrosis.
** Bacterial or viral pneumonia, empyema, pulmonary infarction, TB, RA, SLE, malignancy, pancreatitis.
TP, total protein.

Complications

- Pneumothorax.

- Hemothorax.

- Re-expansion pulmonary edema.

PARACENTESIS

There is no single physical finding that is both highly sensitive and specific for the presence of ascites. The most useful physical findings for making the diagnosis of ascites are a fluid wave, shifting dullness, and peripheral edema. The inability to demonstrate bulging flanks, flank dullness, or shifting dullness are most useful for ruling out ascites.

Indications

- Obtain ascitic fluid for diagnostic tests.

- Decrease respiratory distress and abdominal discomfort caused by ascites.

Contraindications

- Anticoagulation or bleeding disorder (relative).

- Uncertainty if abdominal distention is actually caused by fluid.

- Bowel obstruction or distended bowel.

- Massive obesity (relative).

What to Tell the Patient

A needle will be used to withdraw fluid from the abdomen for diagnosis and/or relief of symptoms. Have the patient empty their bladder before the procedure. **Informed consent is required.**

Equipment

- Paracentesis kit that contains a catheter/needle assembly, three-way stopcock, collection tubing, etc. A thoracentesis kit with the same equipment will also work fine.

- Extra small gauge needles, syringes, and local anesthetic (just in case).

- Appropriate materials to cleanse the skin (if not included in the kit).

- Sterile gloves.

- Mask and goggles.

Procedure

1. Obtain informed consent.

2. Enlist someone else to be your nonsterile assistant (not always necessary but nice to have around).

3. Have the patient lie supine with the head of the bed elevated a bit. Percuss the abdomen to help determine the site for needle entry. Possible entry sites include the midline 3–4 cm below the umbilicus or the right or left lower quadrants midway between the umbilicus and the anterior superior iliac spine (lateral to the rectus abdominus sheath). Avoid old surgical incisions and areas of skin infection.

4. Put on sterile gloves.

5. Cleanse the area and drape the patient.

6. Anesthetize the skin with a 25-gauge needle. Anesthetize the abdominal wall to the peritoneum with a 22-gauge needle. A 20-gauge spinal needle may be used in very obese patients.

7. Advance the catheter/needle assembly (attached to a syringe) through the skin and abdominal wall aspirating along the way, either at an oblique angle or in a ''Z-track'' fashion (once the skin is penetrated, the catheter/needle is moved 1 to 2 cm then advanced further). A small pop may be felt as the needle advances through the fascia.

8. When peritoneal fluid is obtained, slide the catheter into the peritoneal cavity and withdraw the needle. **Never advance the needle back into the catheter.**

9. Attach a 30- to 50-cc syringe with a three-way stopcock to the catheter. If the paracentesis is being done for diagnostic purposes, aspirate the necessary quantity of fluid.

10. If the paracentesis is being done for therapeutic purposes, attach connecting tubing to the sidearm of the stopcock. This may be connected to vacuum bottles or a collection bag. Pump out or allow the vacuum to suck out up to 1 L of ascitic fluid. If the flow of fluid stops, gently manipulate the catheter or reposition the patient. More fluid may be removed from patients with cirrhosis and peripheral edema.

11. Remove the catheter when finished collecting peritoneal fluid.

12. Bandage the site.

13. Write a procedure note, whether or not you were successful.

14. Depending on the clinical situation, samples should be sent for the following: cell count and differential, total protein, albumin, LDH, glucose, specific gravity, Gram's stain, routine culture, fungal stain and culture, and AFB stain and culture. The highest culture yields occur when blood culture bottles are inoculated at the bedside. Greater than 250 neutrophils per microliter is suggestive of peritonitis. Other tests (e.g., cytology, amylase, and triglycerides) may

TABLE 18-3.
ASCITIC FLUID ANALYSIS

Condition	Protein (g/dL)	SAAG* (g/dL)	LDH (IU)	Glucose	WBC (#/cc)	RBC (#/cc)	Amylase
Cirrhosis	<2.5	≥1.1	<200	<60	Low	Low	N/A
CHF	<2.5	≥1.1	<200	>60	Low	Low	N/A
Nephrosis	<2.5	<1.1	<200	>60	Low	Low	N/A
Peritoneal cancer	>2.0	<1.1	>200	<60	High	Very high	N/A
Infection	>2.5	<1.1	>200	>60	Very high	Low	N/A
Pancreatitis	>2.5	<1.1	>200	>60	Variable	Variable	Very high

* Serum ascites albumin gradient (serum albumin-ascitic fluid albumin).

be done as the clinical situation dictates. Refer to Table 18-3 regarding the interpretation of ascitic fluid studies.

Complications

- Persistent ascitic fluid leakage.

- Bowel perforation.

- Hemorrhage.

- Peritonitis.

- Hypotension, oliguria, and shock.

- Bladder perforation.

GUIDELINES FOR OCCUPATIONAL EXPOSURES

- If an exposure to blood or other bodily fluids occurs:

  1. *Stop what you are doing immediately!* Take a deep breath; don't panic.

  2. Cleanse wound with soap and water. For mucous membrane exposures, rinse with copious amounts of water.

  3. Call the hospital's exposure hotline to report the exposure and get further instructions. Each hospital has its own procedures on handling occupational exposures. In reporting an incident, you will need the following information:

     - Date and time of exposure.

     - Details of procedure being performed, amount of fluid or material exposed to, severity of exposure, type of needle used (e.g., hollow bore).

     - Details of exposure source—e.g., known HIV, HBV, HCV positive? If source has known HIV, obtain the names and dosages of medications the source is taking.

  4. You and the source patient will need to be evaluated for HIV, Hepatitis B, and Hepatitis C. Follow instructions from employee/ occupational health for testing and follow-up.

- The risk of transmission of a blood-borne pathogen depends on the pathogen involved, the type of exposure, amount of blood involved in the exposure, and amount of virus in the patient's blood at the time of exposure.

- If you have been exposed, you should avoid exchange of bodily fluids with other persons until follow-up is complete, including using condoms with sexual partners until the results of the HIV test from the source patient are known.

- For more information on postexposure risk and therapies:

  1. National Clinicians' Postexposure Hotline 1-888-448-4911 or http://www.ucsf.edu/hivcntr/PEPline

  2. CDC http://www.cdc.gov/ncidod/hip/Blood/exp_blood.htm

19 Critical Care Notes

... Survival of the fittest ...

KEYS TO INTENSIVE CARE UNIT SURVIVAL

... Always come back to the basics: Air goes in and out. Blood goes round and round. Oxygen is good ...

- Transfer notes (see Chap. 6) with key details of the patient's past medical history and course are always helpful. The primary physician, receiving physician, and the patient's family members should be notified. Note any details or special situations that need attention and/or follow up.

- Admitting a patient to an intensive care unit can be intimidating, but keep in mind the ABCs (Airway, Breathing, Circulation) and focus on stabilizing the patient.

- Be nice to the nurses, respiratory therapists, and other ancillary staff during your stay. They can often make useful suggestions, catch things you miss, and be immensely helpful to you in critical situations. They can be the difference between an enjoyable or miserable experience.

- Ask (and keep asking) if you have questions or problems. Mistakes from inexperience in critically ill patients can have catastrophic consequences.

- Always treat the patient, not the numbers.

- It's always a good idea to make rounds on patients and follow up on labs several times a day even if things seem stable.

- Daily ICU notes should include ventilator settings, I/O's, pulmonary artery catheter measurements, medications and drips (antibiotics, sedatives, pressors), nutritional status, and documentation of every indwelling catheter or tube.

- References to have nearby at all times:

  Winshall J, Lederman R. *Tarascon Internal Medicine and Critical Care Pocketbook*, 3rd ed. Tarascon Publishing, 2004.
  Marino P. *The ICU Book*, 2nd ed. Baltimore: Williams & Wilkins, 1998.
  Kollef M. Critical care. In *Washington Manual of Medical Therapeutics*, 31st ed. Philadelphia: Lippincott Williams & Wilkins, 2004.

VENTILATORS

... Breathe in, breathe out ...

Suggestions for Initial Ventilator Settings
Basic settings

- Mode

  CMV/AC: Guarantees set tidal volume; often best to start with this.
  SIMV + PSV: Choreographed breaths at preselected rate; allows spontaneous breaths.
  PCV: Pressure controlled ventilation; can't guarantee the tidal volume if lung compliance decreases.

- Tidal volume: 10–12 mL/kg versus 5–7 mL/kg in low tidal volume ventilation.

- Rate: 10–15 breaths/minute.

- F_{IO_2}: 1.0, then titrate down (patients should never be ventilated on 100% O_2 >24 hours unless absolutely necessary).

- PEEP: 0–5 cm H_2O (careful with auto-PEEP).

Advanced Settings

(ask for help before you change these)

Inspiratory flow: 50–60 L/min. With COPD may want as high as 100 L/min.
I:E ratio: 1:2. This must be set individually with PCV.
Peak and Plateau pressures: Attempt to keep peak pressure <45 cm H_2O and plateau pressure <35 cm H_2O.

Ventilator Adjustments

- A P_{O_2} of 60 mm Hg or greater is usually the goal. Oxygenation is most affected by mean air pressure. Adjustments to F_{IO_2} and PEEP can help increase oxygenation. Remember that the oxygen saturations tell you nothing about the P_{CO_2}.

- CO_2 is regulated by ventilation. Increasing the respiratory rate or tidal volume blows off more CO_2.

- See Table 19-1 for suggested adjustments.

General "Ballpark" Change Guidelines

- Desired P_{O_2} >60 mmHg. Use this simple ratio to calculate the required F_{IO_2} (defined as X):

$$\frac{\text{Current } P_{O_2}}{\text{Desired } P_{O_2}} = \frac{\text{Current } F_{IO_2} \text{ (\%)}}{X \text{ (\%)}}$$

TABLE 19-1.
SUGGESTIONS FOR VENTILATOR MANAGEMENT BASED ON P_{CO_2} AND P_{O_2}*

	P_{CO_2}	P_{O_2}
High	↑ Minute volume	Decrease F_{IO_2}
	↑ Tidal volume	
	↑ Respiratory rate	
Low	↓ Minute volume	PEEP
	↓ Tidal volume	± Increased F_{IO_2} (in cases of diffusion block, increase F_{IO_2})
	↓ Respiratory rate	

* Individualize for every patient.

(e.g., if P_{O_2} is 150 on 100% O_2 ...)

$$\frac{150}{60} = \frac{100}{X} = 40\%$$

The F_{IO_2} can be reduced to 0.4 and this should maintain a P_{O_2} of 60.

• Desired P_{CO_2}. Another simple formula:

P_{CO_2} (current rate) = desired P_{CO_2} (X)

X = New rate to set to obtain the desired P_{CO_2}

Worsening Oxygenation

The knee-jerk impulse is to turn up the F_{IO_2}. Don't panic, approach the problem in a stepwise manner:

• Is there a ventilator problem?

  • Is the ET tube in the correct position or has it migrated? Check with the nurse on the marking of the ET tube and the most recent x-ray.

  • Is there a cuff leak or kink in the ET tube? Have respiratory therapy check this.

  • Recheck the ventilator settings. Have there been inadvertent changes?

- Is there an obstruction in the ET tube (e.g., mucous plug)? Suction now.

- Is it a patient-related problem (e.g., biting, agitation)? Sedation may be needed.

- Always consider pneumothorax. Listen on both sides and consider a CXR.

- Is the underlying problem worsening? Is the patient fluid overloaded or is there bronchospasm? Is a PE a possibility? Has ventialtor-associated pneumonia developed?

- Is the patient oversedated? Do you need to rethink the mode of ventilation? Check the PEEP level at end-expiration. Hypoxemia can be from a loss of PEEP.

Weaning Parameters

- The method of weaning is not as relevant as knowing the appropriate time to wean. See Table 19-2.

TABLE 19-2.
GUIDELINES FOR ASSESSING WITHDRAWAL OF MECHANICAL VENTILATION

Patient's mental status: awake, alert, cooperative

Po_2 >60 mm Hg with an Fio_2 <0.5

PEEP ≤5 cm H20

Pco_2 and pH acceptable

Spontaneous tidal volume >5 mL/kg

Vital capacity >10 mL/kg

Minute ventilation <10 L/min

Maximum voluntary ventilation double of minute ventilation

Maximum negative inspiratory pressure ≥25 cm H_2O

Respiratory rate <30 breaths/min

Static compliance >30 mL/cm H_2O

Rapid shallow breathing index <100*

Stable vital signs following a 1 to 2 hour spontaneous breathing trial

* Rapid shallow breathing index = Respiratory rate/tidal volume in liters.
From Kollef MH, Critical Care, in *Washington Manual of Medical Therapeutics,* 31st ed. Lippincott, Williams & Wilkins, 2004.

ICU SEDATION

... Sleep tight...pleasant dreams ...

• Ventilated patients generally require sedation. This is usually achieved through continuous IV infusion of sedatives. See Table 19-3.

• Achieve the desired level of sedation with boluses before starting infusion. Level of sedation is commonly measured by the modified Ramsey scale:

LEVEL	PATIENT RESPONSE
1	Patient anxious, agitated, or restless
2	Patient cooperative, oriented, and tranquil
3	Patient asleep, responds to commands only
4	Patient asleep, responds to gentle shaking
5	Patient asleep, does not respond to auditory stimulus, responds to noxious stimulus
6	Patient has no response to firm nailbed pressure or other noxious stimuli

• If the patient becomes agitated, rebolus to desired level of sedation and then make small increments in the drip rate.

• Titrate to minimum effective dose and reasses the need for continuous sedation daily.

• Consider adding paralytics for patients with very poor oxygenation or if agitation persists despite adequate sedation, causing difficulty with ventilation. Make sure the patient is adequately sedated before adding paralytics!

CARDIAC PARAMETERS

... Don't go breaking my heart ...

• Normal cardiac output

5 ± 1 L/min

• Normal cardiac index

3 ± 0.54 min/m^2

TABLE 19-3.
DRUGS FOR ICU SEDATION AND PARALYSIS

Drug	Bolus Dosing	Onset (single dose)	Duration (single dose)	Dilution	Maintenance	Comments
					Continuous infusion	
Fentanyl	50–100 μg	1–2 min	30–60 min	2500 μg/50 mL	50–100 μg/hr; ↑ in 50 μg/hr increments to max 500 μg/hr	Possible bradycardia with bolus doses. Effects prolonged effect in renal and hepatic failure.
Morphine	10–15 mg	5–10 min	3–4 hr	100 mg/100 mL	1–4 mg/hr; ↑ by 2–5 mg/hr to max 50 mg/hr	Possible hypotension. Effects prolonged effect in renal and hepatic failure.
Lorazepam	2–4 mg	20–40 min	3–6 hr	40 mg/40 mL	0.5 mg/hr; ↑ by 0.25 mg/hr to max 4 mg/hr	Effects prolonged effect in renal and hepatic failure.
Midazolam	1–5 mg	1–4 min	30–60 min	50 mg/50 mL	1 mg/hr; ↑ by 1 mg/hr to max 10 mg/hr	Possible hypotension with bolus. Effects prolonged in renal and hepatic failure.
Propofol	0.3 mg/kg (optional)	1–2 min	30 min	1,000 mg/100 mL	25–50 μg/kg/min; ↑ by 10 μg/kg/min to max 100 μg/kg/min	Possible hypotension, bradycardia.
Dexmedetomidine	1 μg/kg over 10 min	10 min	30 min	200 μ/100 mL	0.2–0.7 μg/kg/hr; ↑ by 0.1 μg/kg/hr	Possible hypotension, bradycardia. Do not use for <24 hours.

Adapted from Barnes-Jewish Hospital Guidelines for ICU Sedation and Therapeutic Paralysis. Barnes-Jewish Hospital Department of Pharmacy. St. Louis: Washington University Medical Center, 2004.

- Normal filling pressures

  Right atrial pressure 0–8 mm Hg
  Right ventricular pressure 5–30/0–8 mm Hg
  Pulmonary artery pressure 15–30/3–12 mm Hg
  Pulmonary wedge pressure 3–12 mm Hg

SHOCK

... We're not talking about the electrical kind ...

Hemodynamic profiles associated with shock

	CVP	CI/CO	SVR	SvO_2	PCWP
Hypovolemic (e.g., hemorrhage)	↓	↓	↑	↓	↓
Cardiogenic (e.g., MI, tamponade)	↑	↓	↑	↓	↑
Distributive (e.g., septic)	↓	↑	↓	N - ↑	N - ↓

CVP = central venous pressure; CI = cardiac index; CO = cardiac output; SVR = systemic vascular resistance; SvO_2 = mixed venous oxygen saturation; PCWP = pulmonary capillary wedge pressure; N = normal.

Treatment of Shock

- Determine the type of shock you are dealing with.

- Fluid resuscitation is vital, especially for hypovolemic shock. Crystalloids (normal saline or Lactated Ringer's) should be started immediately. For hemorrhagic shock, blood products should be administered.

- Use of vasopressors and inotropes can be helpful. These are generally titrated to a mean arterial pressure of ≥60 mmHg. Afterload reduction may be helpful in cardiogenic shock. **See Drips section below for dosages.**

DRIPS

... And we're not talking about from your faucet ...

- See Table 19-4 for common drips used in the ICU.

TABLE 19-4.
COMMON DRIPS USED IN THE ICU

	Receptor activity	Dosage	Comments
Vasopressors			
Dopamine	α, β, dopamine	2–3 μg/kg/min for renal and splanchnic dilation (dopamine) 4–8 μg/kg/min for increase in cardiac contractility (β) >10 μg/kg/min for vasoconstriction (α)	Dose-dependent receptor activation
Epinephrine	α, β	Start at 1–4 μg/min, titrate to MAP ≥60	Drug of choice for anaphylactic shock
Norepinephrine	α >β	Start at 2 μg/min, titrate to MAP ≥60	Potent vasoconstrictor
Vasopressin	V1a, V1b, V2	0.04 U/minute	Vasoconstrictor
Inotropes			
Dobutamine	α, β	Start at 3 μg/kg/min, titrate ≤20 μg/kg/min	Has inotropic and chronotropic properties; causes reflex peripheral vasodilation
Milrinone	PDE III inhibitor	0.375–0.75 μg/kg/min	Inotrope, direct peripheral vasodilator
Vasodilators/ Afterload reducers			
Nitroglycerin	Stimulates cGMP production resulting in vascular smooth muscle relaxation	Start at 5–10 μg/kg/min, titrate 10–20 μg/kg/min every 5 minutes until desired effect	At high doses, reflex tachycardia can occur; patients can develop tolerance to medication
Nitroprusside	Direct peripheral vasodilator	Start at 0.25 μg/kg/min, maximum 10 μg/kg/min	Check sodium thiocyanate level with prolonged use; do not use in renal failure

SUGGESTIONS FOR PROPHYLAXIS

... An ounce of prevention is worth a pound of cure ...

- DVT: see DVT prophylaxis section, Chapter 8.

- GI: see GI prophylaxis section, Chapter 8.

- Decubitus ulcers: Turn patient several times a day, vigilant skin care, egg crate mattress or Kin-Air bed, and adequate nutrition.

- Deconditioning: Physical therapy and nutritional support.

- Aspiration precautions: Elevate head of the bed and frequent suctioning (especially around the cuff of ET tube).

- Seizure or fall precautions: as appropriate.

- Infection: Maintain oral hygiene, keep track of lines (IV, NG tube, feeding tubes) and change per protocol, and target or discontinue antibiotic therapy to avoid resistance and *C. difficile* colitis.

- Follow isolation (respiratory or contact) precautions at all times, and wash your hands!

TOTAL PARENTERAL NUTRITION (TPN)

... A viable GI tract is a terrible thing to waste ...

- Consider this option if the GI tract is unusable for at least 7 days. Sterile vascular access is needed.

- Administered through the brown port of the triple lumen catheter. Reserve this port if you think initiating TPN is a possibility—cannot be used if it has been used previously.

- For initial orders and questions, a **nutritional support consult** will be valuable for information, advice, other options, and help with calculating projected nutritional needs.

- TPN orders must be written daily and received by a certain time—make sure this is done before signing out.

- Monitor vital signs, daily weight, I/Os, Accuchecks, and routine labs (CBC, electrolytes, BUN, SMA–9, Mg) frequently. Monitor triglycerides and hepatic function at least once a week.

- May add H_2 blockers, steroids, insulin, and vitamin K to TPN if so desired.

- If TPN must be D/C'ed, monitor Accuchecks and administer IV fluids (e.g., D_{10}) at the same rate.

20   **Final Touches**

... Words to the wise and sleep deprived ...

1. When in doubt, ask and ask again. Call someone (wake up someone if you need to), preferably someone who knows more than you do.

2. When in doubt, it's always better (albeit more painful) to go see the patient.

3. The right thing to do usually involves less sleep.

4. Walk if you don't need to run. Sit down if you don't need to stand. Lie down if there's a bed nearby. Answer all of nature's calls.

5. Take primary responsibility for your patients—you are their doctor.

6. Listen to your patients. They'll usually tell you what you need to know.

7. Resist the temptation to discuss patient care in public areas; no good can come of it.

8. A healthy amount of comparison and compulsion makes it difficult to harm patients.

9. See one, do one, teach one. You'll be expected to assume more teaching responsibilities as time goes on. Start developing your own teaching style and discuss expectations clearly with all learners.

10. Help out your colleagues. If you finish your work early, check with other members of your team or the cross-covering intern to see if they need anything; they can return the favor when you need it most.

11. Before going home for the day, make sure your patients are tucked in and check out with your resident. A complete sign-out is vital—make sure to include any information (studies, consults, procedures) that may be needed to make major therapeutic decisions. Be sure to leave a pager number in case complicated issues arise that need your expertise about the patient.

12. Worthy goals for internship include: learning to distinguish the life-threatening issues from the acute ones from the stable ones; mastering the interpretation and proper usage of diagnostic tests; learning procedural skills; refining the ability to ask specific questions for every consult you request.

13. Fear and anxiety are normal. Take a deep breath and plunge in—there are people around to help you.

14. There is no magic spell on the last day of internship that will turn you into a resident. Trust that if you do and learn the right things during internship, you will be prepared to rise to the challenges of residency.

15. Residency, too, shall pass.

PATIENT DATA TRACKING FORM

Name	
DOB	Age
Admitted	Discharged
Allergies	

HPI

PMH/PSH

Admission Meds

SH   FH

ROS

Admission

T	P	R	BP
O_2		Wt	Ht

MCV=
RDW=

C_A		T bili		PTT				
Mg		D bili		PT				
Phos		AST		INR				
TP		ALT		Amylase				
Alb		Alk Ph		Lipase				

Previous Labs:

EKG   CXR

Admission: Admission:

Previous: Previous:

Previous Studies:

Problems:

Brief Course:

ADMISSION
☐ Old data
☐ Old records
☐ DDx
☐ Admit orders
☐ Interview
☐ H&P
☐ Schedule tests
☐ Read
☐ DVT Proph

DISCHARGE
☐ Placement

☐ Home care

☐ D/C orders

☐ Transport

Date							
Overnight Complaints							
	CP		SOB		CP		SOB	
	N/V		Abd		N/V		Abd	
	Urine		Ap/wt		Urine		Ap/wt	
	Fatigue		BM		Fatigue		BM	
	HA		Vis		HA		Vis	
	Aud				Aud			
Meds							
Relevant Tests							
T (T_{max})							
P							
R							
BP							
SaO2							
I/O							
Accu							
Physical Exam							

Other Labs				
Tasks	□ Pre-round 　□ Notes in chart 　□ Vitals 　□ Meds 　□ Labs 　□ Micro □ Note □ Order tests □ AM Labs	□ Change meds □ Call consults □ Read consults □ Talk with other team members □ Test Results □ Chat with pt and loved ones	□ Pre-round 　□ Notes in chart 　□ Vitals 　□ Meds 　□ Labs 　□ Micro □ Note □ Order tests □ AM Labs	□ Change meds □ Call consults □ Read consults □ Talk with other team members □ Test Results □ Chat with pt and loved ones
A/P				

Index

complications of, 187
contraindications of, 185
equipment for, 185–186
indications of, 185
procedure for, 186–187
Perirectal abscess, 176–177
PICC catheter, guide to use of, 180*t*
Plain abdominal films, radiograph
    interpretation for, 117
Pleural fluid, analysis of, 203–205,
    205*t*
Pneumothorax, 176
Port-a-cath, guide to use of, 179*t*
Positive predictive value (PPV), 19
Pre-excitation syndromes, *96,*
    96–97
Pregnancy, ectopic, 143
Preoperative, risk assessment,
    cardiovascular, 124, 128
Procedure notes, 39–40
Procedures, guide to, 178–210
Prophylaxis
    DVT, 31–32
    GI, 32
    suggestions for, 217–218
Propofol, in ICU sedation, 216*t*
Pruritus, 71
Pseudoaneurysm, femoral artery,
    174
Psychiatric trauma. *See* Domestic
    violence, rape, psychiatric
    trauma,
Psychiatry, consultation for,
    163–170
Psychosis, 166–167
PubMed, 15
Pulmonary disease and allergy,
    Internet resources for, 14
Pulmonary embolism, management
    of, 63
Pulseless electrical activity
    algorithm, *5*
PV. *See* Pemphigus vulgaris

Radial artery, arterial line placement
    in, 198–199, *200*
Radiograph interpretation, 114–122
    for bones, 117
    for chest x-ray, 115–116
    for gastrointestinal structures,
        117–118
    for heart and mediastinum, 116

    for hilar structures, 116
    for lung fields, 116–117
    for plain abdominal films, 117
    for soft tissues, 117
Ramsey scale, modified, 215
Rape. *See* Domestic violence, rape,
    psychiatric trauma
Rash, 71
Red eye (conjunctivitis), 151–153,
    152
Renal failure, acute, workup for,
    50–53
    major causes of, 51
    management of, 52–53
Respiratory acidosis, 112–114,
    113*t*
Respiratory alkalosis, 114, 114*t*
Respiratory rate, as vital sign, 94
Restraints, 164
Reticulocyte count (corrected),
    formula for, 18
Reticulocyte production index,
    formula for, 18
Retinal detachment, 150
Retroperitoneal bleeding, 173
Rheumatology, Internet resources
    for, 14
Right internal jugular vein, central
    venous access in, 191–194,
    192–193
Risk assessment, cardiovascular,
    preoperative, 124, 128
Rounds, in daily assessments, 36
Ruptured globe, 145–146

Second-degree atrioventricular
    block, Mobitz type I, *102,*
    102–103
Second-degree atrioventricular block,
    Mobitz type II, 103, *103*
Seizures, 135–136
Sensitivity, defined, 19
Septic joint, 155–156
Shock
    hemodynamic profiles associated
        with, 217
    treatment of, 217
Shortness of breath, workup for,
    62–64
    causes of, 62
    management of, 63